BY NICHOLAS THOMPSON

The Running Ground: A Father, a Son, and the Simplest of Sports

The Hawk and the Dove: Paul Nitze, George Kennan, and the History of the Cold War

The Baobab and the Mango Tree: Lessons About Development—African & Asian Contrasts (co-author with Scott Thompson)

The Running Ground

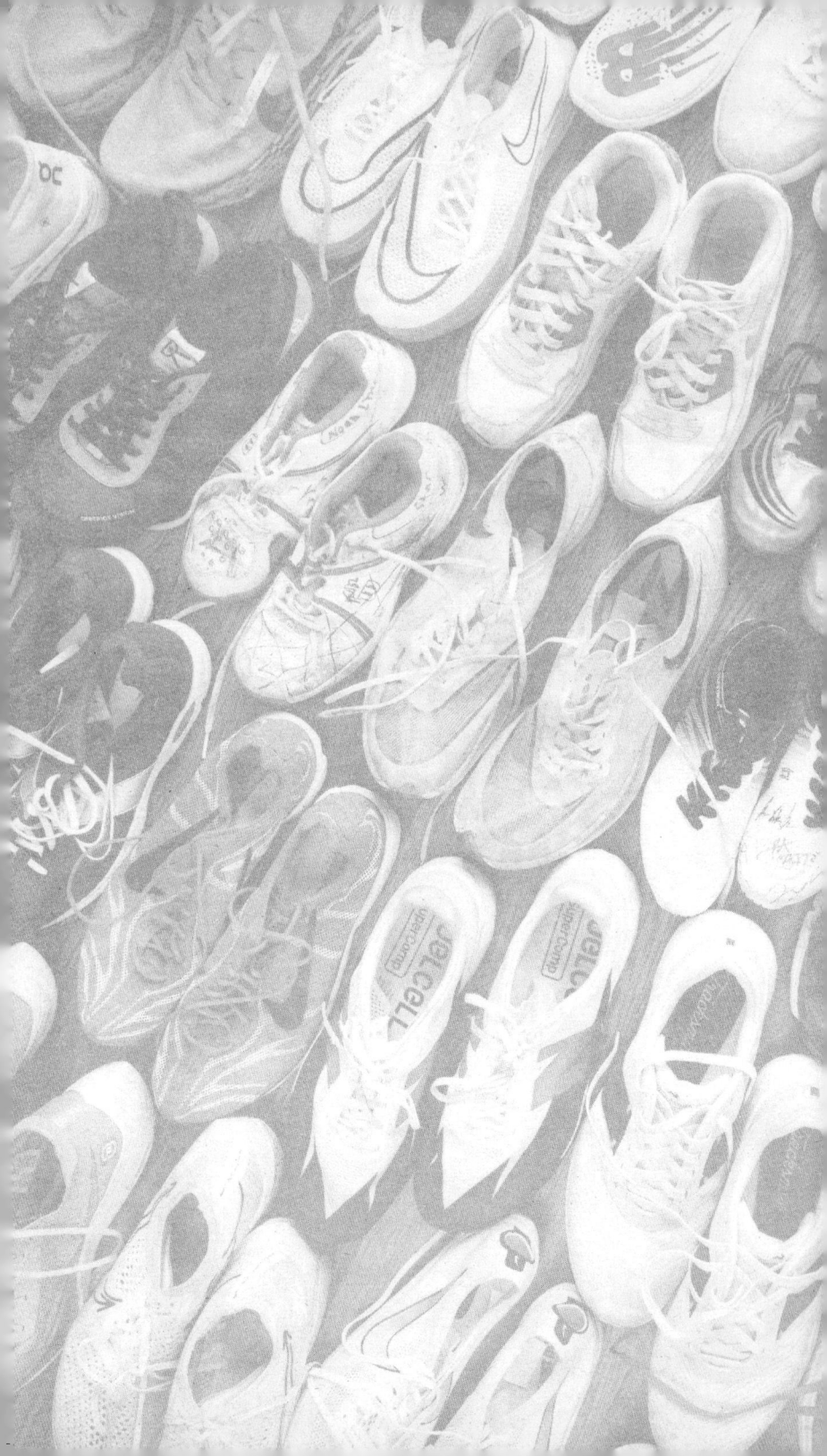

The Running Ground

A Father, a Son, and the Simplest of Sports

Nicholas Thompson

EBURY EDGE

UK | USA | Canada | Ireland | Australia
India | New Zealand | South Africa

Ebury Edge is part of the Penguin Random House group of companies
whose addresses can be found at global.penguinrandomhouse.com

Penguin Random House UK
One Embassy Gardens, 8 Viaduct Gardens, London SW11 7BW

penguin.co.uk
global.penguinrandomhouse.com

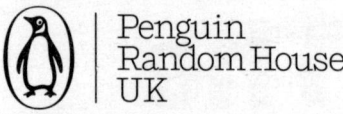

First published in the United States by Random House in 2025
First published in the United Kingdom by Ebury Edge in 2025

1

Copyright © Nicholas Thompson 2025
The moral right of the author has been asserted.

Penguin Random House values and supports copyright. Copyright
fuels creativity, encourages diverse voices, promotes freedom of expression
and supports a vibrant culture. Thank you for purchasing an authorised edition
of this book and for respecting intellectual property laws by not reproducing,
scanning or distributing any part of it by any means without permission. You are
supporting authors and enabling Penguin Random House to continue to publish
books for everyone. No part of this book may be used or reproduced in any
manner for the purpose of training artificial intelligence technologies or systems.
In accordance with Article 4(3) of the DSM Directive 2019/790, Penguin Random
House expressly reserves this work from the text and data mining exception.

Printed and bound in Great Britain by Clays Ltd, Elcograf S.p.A.

The authorised representative in the EEA is Penguin Random House Ireland,
Morrison Chambers, 32 Nassau Street, Dublin D02 YH68

A CIP catalogue record for this book is available from the British Library

Hardback ISBN 9781529146103
Trade paperback ISBN 9781529146110

Book design by Debbie Glasserman

Penguin Random House is committed to a sustainable future
for our business, our readers and our planet. This book is made
from Forest Stewardship Council® certified paper.

To Danielle,
Ellis, Zachary,
and James

Contents

INTRODUCTION xi

CHAPTER 1 **Thirteen Seconds** 3

CHAPTER 2 **Run Around the Block** 14

CHAPTER 3 **Bobbi Gibb** 38

CHAPTER 4 **Just Thanks** 46

CHAPTER 5 **A Tiny Imperceptible Tailwind** 65

CHAPTER 6 **Tony Ruiz** 83

CHAPTER 7 **Falling Apart at Forty** 94

CHAPTER 8 **Julia Lucas** 113

CHAPTER 9 **Here's What's Going to Happen** 122

CHAPTER 10 **Saying Thanks in the Twilight Zone** 135

CHAPTER 11 **Beet Juice** 152

CHAPTER 12 **2:29** 176

CHAPTER 13 **Michael Westphal** 189

CHAPTER 14	**I Wanted to Run a Loop**	196
CHAPTER 15	**Suprabha Beckjord**	206
CHAPTER 16	**A Labrador in a Race for Wolves**	214
CHAPTER 17	**More Than Anything**	230

ACKNOWLEDGMENTS 243
PHOTOGRAPH CREDITS 249

Introduction

RUNNING IS THE SIMPLEST OF SPORTS: RIGHT FOOT, LEFT FOOT, RIGHT foot. There's no ball to focus on, no mat to land on, no one charging toward you with their shoulder down. But the simplicity opens up complexity. As you run, your attention shifts inward. You're just you—right foot, left foot, and whatever goes on in your mind.

Running strips you down. The less clothing you wear, the faster you go. The lighter your shoes, the faster you go. As you go faster, your head empties too. At a certain point, all you can register is the sensation of each foot striking the pavement. Mind and matter briefly become one.

You may have to worry about wind and rain and heat, but

you rarely have to worry about anyone else. You do it by yourself, which gives you control. You don't need to travel to a gym or a field; you just need to open your front door. The sport's simplicity means your successes are your own, and also that there's no one else to blame when you fail. And no sport shows the relentless decline of the aging body more clearly than running. If you can't do what you did a year or a month ago, the evidence is right there on your watch.

Sometimes, I use running as a form of meditation. I put on my shoes and go out. I connect my watch to satellites and then try to disconnect my mind from the swirl inside. Eventually, I'm alone in my head. Sometimes, I'll focus on a musical mantra: "one-two-three, one-two-three," tracking my steps and making sure I keep my left and right feet alternating symmetrically on the downbeat. Other times, I focus on my breath or on the sounds and motion around me, whether the blue jays in the Catskills or the trucks rumbling by on Broadway. Sometimes, as with all meditation, my attention wanders, like a stream flowing haphazardly through my mind, collecting sticks and carrying them until they wash to the side.

When I run a workout, though, everything changes. I'm not trying to open my mind; I'm trying to close it. I shut out the blue jays and the trucks. I have to focus. If I'm with a training partner, I lock my attention on their shoulder if I'm behind or on their breath if I'm ahead. Usually, though, I'm on my own. I look for runners up the road and set imaginary races against them: Can I catch the lady in the purple sweatshirt before the second oak tree? Can I stay an even twenty meters behind the cyclist playing John Coltrane on a boom box? I check my watch and try not to let my pace deviate from the goal. I try to identify the parts of my body that hurt and then I push the pain away from them. I remind myself that I have run this fast before. Self-doubt is a smoldering fire. In a workout, the embers often flash. I don't want to give them any air. Every action we take helps to build our habits. Quit once and it'll be easier to quit the second time too.

I don't listen to music while I run. Every workout is a physical challenge—I'm trying to strengthen the muscles in my legs and my heart—but it's also a mental challenge. I'm trying to teach my body how to move quickly and with good coordination through space. Running is a process of learning about your body and developing habits deep inside it. Music can confuse the signals. I want to deepen my understanding of the relationship between my stride, my pace, my breath. I don't want a bassline, or the adrenaline that can flow with it, to get in the way.

When I race in a marathon, my goal early on is to spend as little energy as possible thinking about anything extraneous. I think about posture and form and balance. I try not to think about the people cheering. I try not to think about past failures or successes. I try to glance as infrequently as possible at my watch. It takes energy, after all, to turn your head, and it takes energy to think. When people in my pack ask questions, or offer commentary, I respond in grunts. On easy runs with friends in the park, I'm a chatterbox. When I race, I'm a vault.

Over the years, the sport has shifted my imagination and my sense of self. When I travel by train, I find myself looking out the window and noting spots to run by the creeks and forests nearby. When I arrive in a new city, I like to circle it with a run. I've seen more of the world while running than I have while walking. I have recurring dreams of mountains I've run up. But I spend much of the day at a desk, mind-wired to my to-do list. Running is my one connection to nature and to a younger, adventurous self who only and always wanted to be outside.

I've always loved the feeling of moving myself fast through empty space. At age five, I ran a mile with my father for the first time. One of my purest childhood memories is of sprinting down the dirt road at my grandparents' farm in Maryland with my sister Phyllis when I was eight and she was nine. We plunged forward, making sure our tiny feet didn't stick in any of the cow grates along the way. Two years later, I beat my mother for the first time in a race from the beech tree near our house to our front door.

In high school, I was adrift and lonely until I stumbled onto the track team. I quickly earned stature and confidence that transferred into the classroom. Realizing I was good at something made me better at everything. I circled the blue track and set school records that helped me get into college. There, the sport taught me about failure, and the cruel idea that you can come up short because you're not good enough, not because you didn't try hard enough.

For the next decade, running was my unrequited crush. I trained like a dilettante and searched for physiological shortcuts that don't exist. I humiliated myself in races. Then, at 29, and in a rut professionally, I started to train seriously again. I found a coach, a team, and my old talent. I started finishing marathons in just a touch slower than 2:40. I wasn't elite, but I was now good enough to win the occasional gift certificate from Dick's Sporting Goods at local road races. I was also old enough to start declining but inexperienced enough to keep improving. For the next decade, these two forces—experience propelling me forward and age pushing me backward—stayed in balance. I was a man walking slowly forward on a moving sidewalk going slowly backward. I ran marathon after marathon in remarkably similar times.

My father had taught me to run, and we had run together for years. The sport was part of his identity. It gave structure to his days, and he viewed it as a sign of vitality. He took pride in everything I did well, but he took a special pride in my running because it was a gift from him. He also warned me many times that my life would fracture at around 40, which was the age at which he'd run his fastest race.

At age 43, my running changed completely. Through happenstance and good fortune, I was connected to a group of elite coaches who asked whether I would be interested in letting them train me for the coming Chicago Marathon. With their help, I started setting personal records. Then, at age 44, I ran a marathon in 2:29, making me one of the fastest marathoners my age in the world. Two years later, I set an American age-group record in the 50K. A few years after that, I became the top-ranked runner in the world in my age group in the 50-mile.

For a long time, I had thought of athletic ability as a mountain. You're born at the base, and you'll die there too. In between, you climb higher and higher until you reach your peak and begin to descend. But as I trained with these new coaches, I began to understand that this analogy isn't quite right, because as you get older you acquire wisdom that can help you get better. Perhaps athletic ability is more like rolling peaks. You go up, you go down. At some point you reach your pinnacle, but there are still vistas as you descend.

I began to see deep connections between my new methods of training and the way I lived and worked. I began to understand the connections between the mental process one uses to run faster and the mental process one uses to get through anything hard. I learned that pain has physical causes but that it's mostly a mental process: we slow in races less because we reach our physical limits than because our minds get scared. I realized that my father was wrong: your life doesn't have to fracture at 40. You can use the lessons you learn in the sport—the discipline, self-awareness, and understanding of life's rhythms—to hold off the kinds of demons that tormented him. I held on tight to running because I came to believe it would both bring me closer to my father and help me avoid becoming him.

This book is partly a story about the mind of one runner. But it's also a book in which I'll tell the stories of five different runners I've met along the way: Bobbi Gibb, Tony Ruiz, Julia Lucas, Michael Westphal, and Suprabha Beckjord. They've all struggled with the sport, and they've all used the sport to process the other ways that life makes us struggle. They show how running can help us both escape and find our way home.

But this is really a story about lots of runners, tying our shoes, heading to the starting line with all the things we carry—in our back pockets and buried deep inside. The gun goes off and we run. We breathe in and we breathe out. We look at the road ahead and step forward with the bodies shaped by what we've done before. We always hurt and we usually finish. We wonder what we just did and why we did it. Then we plan to do it all over again.

I've been racing for 35 years. When I started, I ran two miles in just under 12 minutes. I wanted, then, to run like an adult. This past year, I finished 100 kilometers in the mountains in just over 12 hours. That day, I wanted to run like a child.

Running is the simplest of sports. But if we look closely, it can teach us about the hardest things in life.

The Running Ground

CHAPTER 1

Thirteen Seconds

Never, never, never again take on mice when you can take on tigers. The mice have the right to chew you to death. The tigers will fight and you'll win.

—EMAIL FROM MY FATHER TO ME, DECEMBER 1997

ON A SUNDAY IN EARLY NOVEMBER 2007, I WOKE UP AT 4:30 IN THE morning and tiptoed out of my bedroom, trying not to wake my wife, Danielle. I navigated to the kitchen, using my phone as a flashlight. There I found the breakfast that I'd laid out the night before: bananas and a salt bagel with peanut butter next to a glass of water. I put on my thin, light racing uniform and then draped myself in baggy sweatpants and a sweatshirt from the Salvation Army. I turned the brass knob of our apartment door and headed out into the cool Brooklyn morning, delighted that the house was still quiet. Danielle was sound asleep and nurturing a tiny, curved body—then roughly the size of a blueberry—whose heart had just started to beat.

I was 32 years old, starting my annual pilgrimage from

Brooklyn to Staten Island, where the New York City Marathon begins. From there, it winds through the five boroughs to the finish line in Central Park. On my way to the 4/5 train, I saw other marathoners leaving buildings nearby, like crabs emerging from their burrows in the sand before storming together toward the sea.

Not everyone can run a marathon, but it's remarkable how many can. There are the graceful leaders moving like antelopes on the veldt, and the elite wheelchair racers whose arms are thick as oaks. But then there are the rest of us, of every shape, size, and age. We go to the starting line together before we gradually slip apart. Marathons may be the only sporting event where anybody can directly test themselves against the very best in the world on the same day, in the same place.

I moved slowly down the stairs to the subway, conserving energy by bringing both feet together before moving to the next step. On the 4 train, and then the Staten Island Ferry, I closed my eyes so I could visualize the race. At Fort Wadsworth, where the runners gathered, I lay on my back, stared at the sky, and tried to imagine each mile ahead—but my mind shifted to my father, who had run this race once, in 1982, and ridden the same ferry and sat somewhere in this same park. His life back then was a tempest of contradictions. He was working in the Reagan Administration as he came to terms with the realization that he was gay. He had begun to achieve the professional recognition he had long sought, even as he made a bonfire out of the structures—marriage, family, and social groups—that had supported his career. He had blown up his marriage with my mother and left the leafy Boston suburbs to cruise the alleyways of Dupont Circle.

His life was manic and confused, and he was entering a

period of record-setting promiscuity and little sleep. But he was still a runner, and this habit seemed to create just enough gravitational force for him to hold his life together. He ran every morning, alternating runs of 12 miles and 6 miles. When I visited him at his new home on Q Street, he would head out on a run before I woke up and return, covered in sweat, just as I was making my way down his dusty, half-renovated stairway with its broken banister. On the day of the 1982 New York marathon, he had sat in this park and hit play on Vivaldi's *Orlando furioso* on his Walkman. It was, he would later write, appropriate that he was listening to an opera about "a stirring figure driven mad by the world's demands."

I rubbed Vaseline between my toes to prevent blisters and then made my way to the start at the base of the Verrazzano-Narrows Bridge. I was part of a starting group called "local elite," which sounds more impressive if you focus on the noun and not the adjective. I pulled off my sweatshirt and sweatpants and tossed them to the side. I felt nearly naked in the cold and stood tightly packed with the other runners. We fist-bumped our friends, peed into Gatorade bottles, and waited. I rotated my foot inward and stretched my ankle joint, then eased my ear toward my shoulder to loosen my neck. There aren't that many ways to warm up when pressed shoulder to shoulder with strangers.

Every runner had their reasons to be on the starting line. Each of us had paid $100 or more to shiver in the cold at the start before suffering for hours and getting an apple and a blanket at the end. My reasons were clear. Two years earlier, at the age of 30, I had run this race in 2:43:51, by far my fastest marathon yet. Two weeks later, my doctor found a lump in my throat. I was swept into a series of tests and sent down endless, cold hospital hallways before I learned that I was suffering from thyroid cancer.

The next year was hell. I had my neck sliced open twice; I underwent radiation therapy and lived briefly in isolation. My cancer was eminently treatable, but I was convinced, often, that I was going to die. Danielle and I wanted to have children, but we had to put our plans on hold. How could I bring a new life into this world when the current life was so uncertain? Struggling to understand this cancer, I tried to think of it as a foreign invader, but that wasn't quite right. It wasn't a virus or an infection. It had grown from me, in me. It *was* me.

The announcer called out, "On your marks." I tensed out of habit and leaned forward, putting my weight on the front of my toes. I crossed myself as a reminder that what I was about to do was both spiritual and quite hard. Then the gun fired. "New York, New York" blared from the starting-line speakers, and I was off. Up the bridge we went, looking left to see the skyscrapers of downtown Manhattan, so far north of us now and yet so far south of the finish line in Central Park. The bridge swayed ever so slightly as the mass of runners began to storm across.

I followed precisely the plan I had for the race, running calmly down into Bay Ridge, Brooklyn. These were quiet miles, with people strolling out to the side of the course with their signs and Sunday-morning coffee. I ran with my friend Corey, drafting, or taking turns blocking the wind, as we moved down the thoroughfare of Fourth Avenue and past its mix of bodegas and nineteenth-century churches. I was once told that a runner begins a race with a hundred pennies of energy in his or her pocket. The goal is to spend those pennies as evenly as you can until, in a sprint at the end, you drop the last one. In these first few miles, though, it's easy to waste pennies: high-fiving a random spectator on the side or accelerating slightly to get around someone in your way. I started to keep track of the runners going at my pace and gave them names in my head. There was "yellow singlet," "purple shorts," "hairy back." I analyzed their posture and the sound of their breath.

With each step, I tried to visualize a different part of my body, moving with strength and relaxation. I thought about my toes pressing through my soft socks, onto the foam of my racing shoes, onto the hard asphalt and then pushing me off. I concentrated briefly on the sensation in my calf and my Achilles tendon: the force going down and then propelling me forward. I marveled, as I often do, about how strange it is that one spends roughly half of each race suspended in air. I imagined a straight line up my back from my sit bones to the base of my skull, a balloon attached to my head, keeping me upright and balanced. And I worried about all the silly things that runners worry about: Were my contact lenses going to slip out of place? Had I put on enough sunblock to prevent a burn but not so much that it would make it harder to sweat? If I had a slight sensation that I was going too fast or too hard, I looked at my watch. If my pace was too fast, I would breathe in through my nose and out through my mouth, relaxing my body and trying to bring in a sense of calm.

Sometimes, my mind drifted. Deep in a race, lost in desperate agony, you want to disassociate and send your mind off into the clouds. Part of learning to race, though, is learning how to lock back in. Focus on the shoes of the man ahead of you; focus on your breath; focus on your feet. Meditate on the task at hand. Disassociation usually makes you slow.

After 44 minutes, we neared my favorite spot of the whole race: mile seven, where Danielle would emerge from Union

Street in Park Slope, Brooklyn. Several blocks before that, I moved out of my pack to the right side of the road so that she'd be able to spot me. She stepped out of the crowd, and I stepped toward it and kissed her on the cheek. I thought about the child who might appear in seven or eight months. I thought back to two years earlier, when she had waited at the very same spot as I ran toward her with an unknown poison growing in my neck.

When you have cancer, there are many hard moments: meetings with doctors, phone calls with results, treatments, scans, surgeries. I can remember the feel of the sweater I was wearing when I got one particularly discouraging call from my doctor, and the cold floor of our bathroom where I once lay vomiting endlessly after a round of treatment. But now I remembered a cold afternoon on Union Street just a few blocks uphill from the racecourse. I was done with my treatments and the scar on my neck was starting to heal. I walked out of our fourth-floor apartment and turned right on Eighth Avenue and then right again on Union Street, eager to walk the slightly uphill block that would take me into Prospect Park. I had lost much of my strength and was walking slowly, effortfully. One foot and then the other. But I couldn't do it. I stopped at a house about halfway up the block and sat on the bottom step of its stoop, dizzy and disoriented, weakened by my medications. I couldn't even walk around the block. Would I ever be able to race again? I kept trying, though—going a little farther every day. Eventually, my strength returned. First, I could walk up the block, then I could run it. Then I could run around the park. And here, in November 2007, I was back out on the course, running at the same pace I had in November 2005.

After kissing Danielle, I turned right on Lafayette Avenue, passing the Brooklyn Academy of Music where a jazz band played. Every so often, I glided out of my pack at a water station to grab a paper cup, like a starling briefly breaking from its flock. Then on to Williamsburg, passing the Hasidim in their furry shtreimels. I felt the slightest of pains at random moments. The top of my left knee hurt for a minute. An old injury in my right iliotibial band made itself known. But these were the nips of a mosquito, not the bites of a lion that I expected to come. I saved precious seconds by running on the crown of the road, the flattest part, and, when all other factors were equal, choosing the shadier side of the course. I had practiced running in a perfectly direct line countless times: watching my right or left shoe land with the edge directly on the white traffic line on a road. Now I would do that while I followed a practice of "running the tangents," looking to the horizon and running the straightest route I could, shaving precious meters off the total distance I would have to cover.

We left the bustle of Brooklyn and crossed the Pulaski Bridge over Newtown Creek, the contaminated tributary that marks the border between Brooklyn and Queens and the exact halfway point of the race. I wondered why the bridge seemed so steep on the way up and nearly flat on the way down. At about mile 14.5, someone on the sideline screamed "almost halfway there," which should have led to their immediate arrest. These were hard miles, and my mind started to drift in the quiet of Queens. I started to do calculations about how much I could slow and still run a decent time. I wondered if, ethically, I could be proud of doing well since it made each person behind me finish one place worse. My mind wandered for about two minutes before I snapped myself back. No, I was here. I had a goal. I was going to run faster than I had two years before. I looked for Corey and "purple shorts" and slowly caught back up.

We rounded onto the Queensboro Bridge. It's darker, and much quieter, than everything before. There's nobody cheering, no sounds of the city. I climbed up to the crest and passed the marker for mile 15. Then I descended, hitting mile 16, and heard the crowd roar like the sound in a ballpark when the hometown slugger hits a deep drive to left. Loud, louder, louder still. I came down and saw the beautiful blue-and-white tiles embossed near the base of the bridge. I felt like a human cannonball, flying out toward the circus crowd.

It was here that, twenty-five years earlier in 1982, I had stood with Florrie, my Irish Catholic nanny, and searched for my father in the sea of sweaty people in short shorts at mile 16. The leaders blitzed by, and he wasn't with them. Then the trickle of runners became a stream and then a river. I worried that we had missed him. But thirty minutes after the leaders, my father ran down the bridge. He must have seen me before I spotted him because I remember him swinging out of the pack toward me. I remember the sweat on his hairy shoulders, and I remember a sense of love that emanated from him. I handed him a bottle of orange juice and gave him a fresh pair of New Balance shoes. He bent down on one knee, almost in prayer, tying the knot. He finished, smiled, and hurried onward.

My father's goal that day in 1982 had been to finish in under three hours, and he came close, missing by only a minute. I didn't then have much sense of how the sport worked—or, for that matter, how fatigue or time worked—and for years, I would wonder why he hadn't just sprinted at the end.

I held on to this image—of my father at the bridge—before shifting to focus on my own stride and my breath. I was feeling confident, and my pace was still good. I felt a dull weight across my body, though, and I could tell that I was starting to slow. I reached the Willis Avenue Bridge, which takes you into the Bronx. As I started that little climb, something started to feel just a bit off-center. There's a distinct feeling I get in a race or a workout when I've done just a little too much or gone just a little too fast. It's not a sharp pain like stepping on a nail or even having a stone in my shoe. When it starts, it's not even physical: there's just a heaviness or dizziness that sets in. Gradually, if it's a bad day, as it was today, the pain spreads, radiating through my body. I started to lose my hand-eye coordination. I reached for a water cup and spilled it on my right calf. I tried to grab another and missed it completely.

By the time I hit mile 21 and entered Harlem, my brain was hosting a *Crossfire*-style debate about my body. On one side, there was a Nick, standing tall and proud, urging me on. *Keep the pace. Five miles to go. You can go faster than you went before you got sick.* Across the dais, a different Nick, somewhat haggard, was making the case to slow, just for a minute. *Wouldn't it be great to just relax a bit? You could breathe in, rest, smile at all these lovely people on the side. You've done a lot already; coming back from cancer is hard. That little sensation in the knee? That one in the lower back? It might be something serious that will haunt you for years.*

The confident voice prevailed. I passed Marcus Garvey Park at mile 22. I had visualized myself here, strong as a gazelle and ready to glide into Central Park, but that wasn't to be. Runners were now overtaking me. I thought of how hard it had been to get fast again after being sick. Running with speed isn't just a physiological process: it's a psychological one. You have to remember what it feels like to pump your arms and legs at a rapid cadence in sync. You have to remember how to make yourself run once or twice more up that hill that you don't want to run up anymore. I had spent years learning these skills, and then a clump of cells in my neck had forced me to learn them all again.

The course enters Central Park at East 90th Street, just before the marker for mile 24. By now my mind was almost empty. I was still moving forward, but I thought of nothing except the step ahead and the sensation that would ricochet through my body when my foot hit the ground. These were miles on the course I had run hundreds of times. Friends stood along the sidelines cheering my name or taking photographs that they would later send me. But I didn't hear or see them. At the end of a race, your peripheral vision shuts down.

Finally, I could see the finish and a familiar time displayed on the clock above. I started to sprint as best I could. I crossed the line in 2:43:38, 13 seconds faster than I had run before I got sick.

We get through most days in life without having to really think about death, which also means that we don't spend a lot of time dwelling on the remarkable fact that we are alive. But sometimes, we feel love, or danger, nearby. There's a boulder crashing down the crevasse we're hiking. Maybe it's heading right toward us; maybe it has just missed us and is now thundering through the forest below. And then, no matter where we are—an actual mountaintop, our childhood bedroom, or the delirious finish of the New York City Marathon in Central Park—our eyes and minds open. We kiss the ground and praise whatever god we worship for putting us in this place, at this time.

My eyes filled with tears as I looked at my watch, saw my time, and realized what I had just accomplished. Then I wrapped myself in a shimmering space blanket, grabbed an apple and a bottle of water, and hobbled forward to exit the park. I headed down to the train that would take me home and sat on the brown wooden bench on the platform. An elderly man in a parka asked how I had done. "I did great," I responded with a smile. He nodded and I had a sense that he understood precisely what I meant: that I had pushed through something terrifying in life and come out on the other side just a bit stronger. He'd made it to an age where he'd probably had moments like this too. I got onto the train and began the trip home, south and under the city. In a little while, my train would pass deep underground, beneath thousands of marathon runners still heading north toward the finish line.

CHAPTER 2

Run Around the Block

If you can fill the unforgiving minute
With sixty seconds' worth of distance run,
Yours is the Earth and everything that's in it,
And—which is more—you'll be a Man, my son!

—RUDYARD KIPLING, "IF—"

MY FATHER BEGAN TRAINING FOR MARATHONS DURING THE GREAT running boom of the 1970s. In 1980, I started tagging along. My father plotted out a mile by driving his Volkswagen Scirocco, eye on the odometer, around the block where we lived, just outside Boston. Start at the front door by the boxwoods, turn left and left again. Go two full loops around the block, and, on the third, stop at the gate in the fence just past the beech tree. The block was in a beautiful suburban oasis, but it had a touch of violence. Each time we rounded the northeastern corner, we had to pass a pair of enraged German shepherds, fenced in but menacing as they tracked us. Then it was back to the quiet chestnut trees and Tudor-style houses. I remember the triumph of running the whole thing by my father's side. Running a full mile made me feel as though I'd done something real. I proudly placed my tiny sneakers next to his size-nine shoes by the front door.

In the back of that house with the boxwoods, we had a long, beautiful garden, and at the far end was a yew bush. You could duck in there during a game of hide-and-seek and be completely invisible. I would play in the leaves with my father and my older sister, Phyllis, and then we would all do pushups while my mother cared for my newborn sister, Heidi, inside. Under his bed, my father kept a red 10-pound weight that he used for sit-ups, and sometimes I would sneak in and try to use it too. When I picture him now, I see him as he was in 1980, 38, strong and smiling, and running in his red Lacoste shirt with socks that could stretch to his knees but were squished down at his ankles.

For the most part, my childhood was blissful, even after my father moved away in 1982. My mother sent me to a lovely private school in Brookline, Massachusetts, where I joined the math team, sang the patter song in *Iolanthe,* and built a giant stereo cabinet in shop class. I adored my sisters. The walls in our handsome brick house were lined with books. I had a yard and a basketball hoop. The banister never broke. I went to church every Sunday and donned a blue blazer when I traveled on an airplane. I spent my time putting together puzzles and creating games with my *Star Wars* figurines. My mother drove me to endless soccer games and tennis tournaments. She took me to ice hockey practices at 5 A.M. She read me stories every night, often nodding off in her chair as I fell asleep.

My mother's parenting style was to provide a remarkable degree of freedom and independence, within a couple of crucial restraints. She would draw boundaries around wherever we were and then let me roam freely within them. "We made a deal when you were little," she would often say years later. "I could dress you in whatever I wanted you to wear, and then you could do whatever you wanted to do."

My mother was a single parent, with three kids, whose ex-husband was a tornado. When he left, he ransacked the home they shared and, shortly thereafter, decided to make a sport of filing custody lawsuits against her on Mother's Day or her birthday. At one point, he called my grade school and falsely reported that a man was coming to kidnap me. Throughout all this, my mother decided to earn a PhD and start a career as an art historian. She volunteered every Sunday at our church. Her friends bequeathed her at least twenty-five godchildren. I never saw her crack.

My father complained about my mother endlessly, but my mother almost never mentioned him. Fifteen years after my father left, she married a litigator from Ropes & Gray. My sisters and I adored him, and my mother found a calm she'd never had with my father. She built a lighthouse for us in the stormy seas that my father stirred up. The qualities of "patience" and "endurance" are so similar that they are the same word in Greek, *hypomonē*. As the apostle Paul wrote, "We rejoice in our sufferings, knowing that suffering produces endurance, and endurance produces character, and character produces hope." I think my mother could have been an excellent marathoner.

My sisters and I would see our father once a week for dinner in Brookline, and we'd journey to Washington, or to his farm in Warrenton, Virginia, for occasional weekend and summer trips. My father's central project was to keep my two sisters and me—but particularly me—from going soft. He resented the world I grew up in and worried that we would emerge from our

Brookline private school without calluses on our hands. He had grown up in Oklahoma and left to join the New England elite. Now he wanted to put a little Oklahoma into his New England elitists.

He gave us lists of chores—sweep by the pool, mow the lawn—which he'd put on the fridge, and gave us 25 cents for finishing each one. He taught me to rotate the tires on the car and to drive a tractor. We dug huge fire pits to burn our garbage and spent weeks planting poplar trees all along the driveway. My sisters and I painted all the rooms inside the house. Every summer, we stained the outdoor porch and pulled out the nails that had popped up in the Virginia humidity. He paid me $10 to read *A Tale of Two Cities* when I was in the sixth grade. Phyllis, then in seventh, had to read *Anna Karenina*.

I never resented the work. He admired productivity, and he paid attention to us when we were being productive. He'd tell me stories as we yanked on the bolts of his Mitsubishi or painted the walls. If I identified the aria of a Mozart opera, he would tell me all about Mozart's childhood. Every now and then, he and I would put on our worn-down sneakers, yell for the dogs, and run a mile or two down the Virginia roads.

There were still clouds. For three years, my father dated a man I'll call Jack who stole statues and paintings from auction houses. He intentionally ran his car over my older sister's cat, and he tried to drug my dog to death. (My resilient dog survived; he got his revenge one morning by running upstairs and defecating in their bed.) Jack once dragged me across the kitchen by my legs in a way that he pretended was playful but that hurt like hell. He pulled a knife on a babysitter. His only virtue was his frequent absence. My father feared that Jack would murder him in the hopes of getting a life insurance payout. So he adjusted his will to leave Jack just three things: a copy of M. Scott Peck's *People of the Lie,* Hobbes's *Leviathan,* and a large dildo.

In the summer when I was eleven, my father, my sisters, and I spent most of our time at the creek, trying to build a swimming hole. This wasn't a simple project: we needed logs, mud, and hundreds of rocks. Phyllis, Heidi, and I would stand with my father in the muddy waters, shoveling mud and flicking it on top of the rock pile. He would carry big rocks from upstream and yank at fallen trees. We'd slowly patch the dam together and watch the river widen. Then we'd take shovels and dig deeper. Every day, we'd arrive to find a new hole in the dam. But eventually, we could swim under water, at least for a few feet. My father would dive down, playfully dunking us, before emerging with instructions on the next rocks to haul.

■

My father's father, Frank Thompson, came from a line of homesteaders, ranchers, and gun-slinging explorers of the American West. Frank was born in 1909 and grew up in a poor, sparsely populated patch of the Verde Valley in Arizona. Many days, he walked seven miles to join the other 100 students at Clarkdale High School. Eventually, he moved to California and became the first person in his family to make it to a college of any sort, attending the University of Redlands. He didn't know how to dress, and he didn't have any money, but he was a sportsman. He became a Golden Gloves champion and he ran the half-mile for the track team. He also could debate. The campus newspaper, in the fall of 1933, reported on a competition with another young man who went on to have a noteworthy career. "Frank Thompson, a prominent junior in campus speaking circles, placed second in the Southern California extemporaneous speaking contest held in the Student Body Auditorium at Whittier College. Richard Nixon of Whittier was the first-place winner."

After college, Frank decided that he had been called by God to become a missionary. He believed that he was one-sixteenth Sioux, and he became a librarian at Bacone College, a Baptist school for Native Americans in Muskogee, Oklahoma. He fell in love with a young singer and music instructor from Missouri named Loretta Long. They married in 1939, my aunt Sara Sue was born in 1940, and my father, Willard Scott Thompson, arrived on New Year's Day, 1942. Frank attended seminary in New England, became a minister, and then returned to Bacone as the school's president.

My father grew up terrified of his father. In an unpublished memoir, he wrote, "The problem was simple; I was not the son my father wished. He would give me geometrically increasing incentives to do push-ups, pull-ups or anything athletic. He was generous in his gift of baseball bats, footballs, finally resigning himself to archery. I sensed his rejection in a variety of ways." My father was uncoordinated and athletically indifferent. He wanted to listen to Bach and Mozart. As an adult, he would claim, implausibly but tellingly, that his first full sentence was, "Mother, put on the *Eine kleine Nachtmusik*." At school, he was the academic star. At home, he would hide behind a curtain and read, fearing that his father would demand he go outside to play baseball.

The family fell apart, my father writes, after his beloved sister, Sara Sue, began a relationship with a glamorous young painter named Dennis Belindo. She was 14 and Belindo was an 18-year-old freshman at the college. Frank was livid and embarrassed. "This was conservative Oklahoma in the 1950s," my father's closest childhood friend, Rick West, told me. "Young men who did that ended up in ditches out in the country."

Frank had already grown weary of the constant fundraising. Now he felt he had to resign his job because of the scandal. "From that point there was nowhere to go but down," my father wrote in his memoir. Frank was only 46 years old, but his drinking picked up and he never recovered his professional stature. To my father, the family never felt intact again. Frank spent the next 25 years striving for a job of equal prominence and purpose. He became a minister and a pacifist activist. But he never felt fully professionally fulfilled.

My dad escaped his unhappy home after reading in *Time* magazine about the oldest incorporated boarding school in America, a place called Phillips Academy in Andover, Massachusetts. He won a scholarship to summer school and started a newspaper, which he used as an excuse to interview faculty members, particularly ones who might have a say in the admissions process. By September, he had an offer to attend as a regular student and a scholarship for $1,050 out of the $1,300 tuition. When Frank declared that the remaining $250 was too much of a burden on the family, my father pulled out a bank statement showing his earnings from a paper route he'd done on horseback and a small gardening business he'd begun. My father later wrote, "This may sound gratingly superficial now, but I was born with the belief, or inculcated into it, if there's something better than I have, I should go for it."

Andover wasn't easy. He showed up with the wrong clothes and was woefully far behind academically. He was picked on, belittled, and, when the seasons turned, pelted with snowballs.

In his memoir, he wrote, "For the first time I not only wasn't a winner, I was a big loser." But, he added, "I learned one thing from my father, who was a champion boxer. When you're knocked out or knocked down, what you did was to get up." He used a safety razor to cut the pockets off his shirts, making them look more like the ones from Brooks Brothers that the other boys wore. He studied harder than all the affluent kids from private schools and earned a reputation on campus for being the last one to turn off his lights at night. His grades went from among the worst in the class to among the very best, and he earned the grudging respect of the popular, athletic students on campus by teaching them how to identify symphonies to help them pass their music classes. When George Kennan, the diplomatic sage and former ambassador to the Soviet Union, came to campus, my father guided him around. He won a $200 academic prize. He put the money in the stock market, where it grew almost twenty-fold before his father, without asking, sold it to pay off his medical bills.

My father gained confidence by joining the cross-country team. He didn't race, but he would run breezily through the bird sanctuary with the other runners. "I didn't have to compete directly," he wrote in his memoir, "and I got better with every run. No longer could I be humiliated in competitive sports arenas." He added that "I found myself in a worthy group of superior young gentlemen, all better off than I, all more experienced, but all amused by my determination."

Later in life, as he worked his way into the Eastern establishment, my father mostly viewed his heritage as something to conceal. But wherever he went, he carried a painting from his childhood. It was of a Native American man in a full-feathered headdress playing a drum. He had placed it above my childhood bed in Boston. After the divorce, Dad took it and then carried it with him from Virginia to Indonesia and then to the Philippines, where he lived in his 60s and 70s. It was one of the objects he held most dear.

A few years ago, I called up Rick West. I sent him a photograph of the painting. "Oh," said West, "that's the work of Dennis Belindo." My father had kept with him a reminder of the world he had lived in before—and perhaps of the fight he thought had broken his father. Sometimes we hold objects tight because they remind us of love; sometimes we hold objects tight because they remind us of pain. I used to think that my father had hung this in my room because he wanted me to have a symbol of masculine strength, of music, and of his roots. Now I realize it was likely something deeper. I can only surmise. But I have to suspect that, even when I was just five years old, he was trying to tell me something about the things in the world that can break a man.

■

My father told me throughout my childhood that Andover was the best high school in America. My mother certainly wasn't going to object. It was just forty-five minutes from home, and it had a beautiful art museum filled with Cassatts and Whistlers. I applied and got in. She drove me up with my suitcases, moved me into my dorm room, and gave me a philodendron to keep by the window. As in all things in my life, my father wanted me to excel and to win. My mother wanted me to be true to myself, content, and kind to others. I was leaving home for the first time, and, appropriately enough, her parting gift was a plant that can survive in any light.

I started Andover in the tenth grade. During my first semester, I was lonely and awkward. My grades were mediocre, and I struggled to find friends. I was 15 and pimply, and through a quirk in the housing system, I'd been placed in a dorm for eight people, six of whom were post-graduates who had already finished high school somewhere else. Once I was quietly preparing for a biology test in a common room when I heard one of them—a star on the football team—start making out with a female teacher I knew well against the other side of the door to the kitchen. I was trapped and had to wait for them to finish before I could sneak back upstairs.

In that winter of my sophomore year, though, I became suddenly fortunate through what seemed like misfortune. I had been captain of my grade-school basketball team, but I was quickly cut from tryouts for the Andover varsity and then, to my chagrin, both the junior varsity and the junior-junior varsity. Sophomores were required to play sports, and indoor track was the one team still accepting castaways. I told the coach I wanted to join.

I had the look of a distance runner: tall and lanky with neither the shoulders to throw nor the quads to jump. The coach told me that I should run the two-mile and that our first meet would be in a week. I trudged out in the shoes I'd worn to math class and did reasonably well, completing the twenty-one and a half loops around the oval in just under 12 minutes. My time put me right about average for boys and right near the star girl on the team, Chrissy Bergren, who ran with long blond pigtails reaching all the way down her back.

Gradually, my curiosity and my intensity developed. I noticed that I had at least a drop of talent. I also didn't have anywhere to hide. An indoor track race is an inverse aquarium: everyone is on the inside looking out at you as you run your laps. I began to pay close attention to the drills and the stretches and to study the better runners. The captain was a senior named Brian Mendonca, who was also president of the student newspaper. There was Lex Carroll, a charismatic senior and 1000-yard runner who also starred on the soccer team. There was a lanky senior named Mike Blanton who wanted to break 10 minutes for the two-mile. He was an honors student and an aspiring physicist. I started to improve, which made me believe that one day I could be like these guys: smart, confident, slightly weird, and very fast.

Toward the end of the season, I ran the two-mile in 11:34 and stood at the finish, upper body bent forward, hands on my sides, heaving. Blanton, who had finished more than a minute earlier, came by to congratulate me. I told him I had gone as fast as I possibly could. He smiled and said to just keep training.

My coach, too, saw potential. The next race was the New England Prep School Championships, and each school was allowed to enter two runners for each event. I doubted he would choose me. Blanton would get one of the spots and then there were two seniors who had also run around 11:30. But the coach had a hunch that I might swallow a lightning bolt. So, on a magical day in February 1991, at a school in Providence called Moses Brown, I was sent to the starting line of the most important race I had ever run. I worried I would come in last. Blanton told me to just relax and run. I warmed up with him and then deferentially moved behind the runners crowded at the start.

I had planned the race precisely. I had run enough on the Andover track to know exactly the lap splits I needed to run a 5:45 mile and thus an 11:30 for the two-mile. What I didn't know, wasn't told, and somehow didn't realize was that the Moses Brown track had a slightly different size and shape.

Someone yelled "Go!" and off we went. I watched the back of Blanton's jersey as he moved into the lead. I felt strong and crossed the first lap in exactly the time I wanted. After the second lap, I was still right on target. Somehow, I was near the best runner from our rival school. He was expected to finish in around 11 minutes. Maybe, I thought, he was having a bad day.

When I passed the one-mile mark, someone yelled out "Five twenty-four, five twenty-five," which I found bewildering. Had they miscounted the laps? I figured there had been an error, but the only thing to do was to keep running. I glided along, blissfully unaware of just how fast I was going and just how tired I ought to be. Something was going well, because my teammates were screaming in a way they never had before, and I kept passing people. I sprinted to the line and looked at the clock. I had finished in third place in a class-record time of 10:48. I stood, on the side of the track, astonished, in my sweaty dark-blue singlet and short white shorts. My coach and teammates ran up to congratulate me, smiling with wonderment and respect. I had been no one, and now I was someone.

Setting a sophomore record in a distance race in a second-tier sport didn't make any girls swoon. But now I had an identity. The football star read about it in the school paper and congratulated me. Blanton, who had run 40 seconds faster and won the race, gave me an "Andover Cross Country" T-shirt that had been passed down for years from the fastest senior to the fastest underclassman.

I learned something from that track at Moses Brown, something I've come back to countless times in my life. If I had understood how fast I was running, I wouldn't have been able to run that fast. Because I didn't know the track, because I didn't know how long the laps were, I didn't get scared and shut down my body. I just kept going. To do it, I had to first forget that I couldn't do it.

A week or two later, I charged down Salem Street with Mendonca. We were wrapping up a workout that had taken us to a beautiful spot called Holt Hill, and the setting sun reflected gently off the snow piled up on the sides of the road. The two of us were in the road, not on the sidewalk. We weren't exactly racing, but we also weren't not racing. We were trying to go as hard as possible without making it seem like we were trying to win. I was side by side with him, my skinny sophomore legs matching his muscular senior strides. I breathed in the cold air and pushed. I tried to quiet my panting. We were going at a blissful, perfect speed, with the tachometer on the red line but not past it. Mendonca seemed surprised I was keeping up.

■

I was eager to talk about my new success with my father, who visited me nearly every week that year. He was thrilled that I was becoming a runner and that I was starting to have confidence in myself.

He commuted up to Boston to teach international politics at Tufts on Mondays. When class was done, he'd zoom up to Andover and meet me at my dorm, often carelessly dressed in a suit that didn't quite fit, a collared shirt that was never buttoned at the top, and socks with holes in them. He was shorter than

I—5'9" versus 6'1"—with thin hair on his head and a bald spot that he'd fought a losing battle against for years. He had blue eyes that my sisters and I always envied, and crow's feet beneath them that we knew would come for us too. He was lean and always darting about: more a squirrel than a lion. But he had a firm handshake, and he'd always grip my hand as though he was trying to squeeze the pulp from a grapefruit. "A man should shake hands like a man," he'd say. I'd smile and try to squeeze back, but it wasn't a skill I practiced much. Then we'd head off to dinner at Pasta Villaggio.

Driving with my father felt like strapping yourself into the Twisted Timbers rollercoaster at Kings Dominion park. Every time he neared the crest of a hill, he'd accelerate; he also believed, contrary to physics and lived experience, that one gained control by accelerating around corners. He thought all other drivers were idiots; if he saw a car that was about to leave a parking space, he'd swerve up to it, put on his blinkers, and then denounce the other driver if he had to wait more than a second or two. They were, he'd say, doing their nails to annoy him or just wasting time to make him mad. I was in the car at least four times when he collided with other vehicles. Once, my father, believing the other driver was at fault, got out of the car to confront the driver, who immediately sped off. My father jumped back into our car and gave chase, hurtling through red lights as though we were in *The French Connection*. I gripped the side of the door and double-checked my seatbelt. Mercifully, the other car got away before anyone was bent around a lamppost.

On those Monday nights in high school, we'd careen into whatever spot was available, and he'd be out the door and walking toward the restaurant before I'd unbuckled my seatbelt. We'd order fettuccine alfredo, and then he'd report on whatever he had observed in his few seconds of seeing me while he picked me up. He told me—correctly—that my friend Todd would come out of the closet in a year or two. He noted—correctly again—that my girlfriend Liz would eventually come out of the closet too. In the middle of my sophomore year, I was working on a paper and complained that although I'd written four drafts, it still wasn't good. He responded, "Well then, write five, or ten, or twenty." He had been behind too, he reminded me, when he started at Andover, and he'd caught up by outworking everyone else. I listened. By my junior year, I had become one of the most focused students on campus.

These were years when I admired my father easily. He had read all the books I was reading and spoke with confidence about everything that mattered to me. One of his great virtues as a professor, and a parent, was his ability to engage and listen. Often he disagreed with me, but he didn't condescend. He'd hear me out and ask questions. Eventually, the check would come, and my father would complain that the waiter was wasting time to annoy him. He'd leave a skimpy tip and pocket the pen as revenge. Then he'd be off at full speed back to the car.

■

After my triumph at Moses Brown, I was hooked. I dropped spring tennis for spring track and continued to model myself after the senior runners. At graduation, Lex Carroll won the school's highest honor: the Aurelian Honor Society Award, given to the student who most exemplified character, leadership, and scholarship. My father had spoken of the award with reverence. He hadn't won it, but he wished he had.

The next fall, I dropped soccer for cross country. I was growing my hair long, and I had to hold it back in a painter's cap. I remember lining up on the great green lawn behind the art museum, in a soft white singlet and blue shorts. I wore light-blue racing shoes with yellow flowers that I had painted on the toes. The race would start, and I would dash across the lawn and then down around the chapel. I'd race past the yellowed stone of Stowe House, where Harriet Beecher had lived while writing essays for the first issues of *The Atlantic Monthly*. I'd cross the heavy grass under the chestnut tree by Rabbit Pond, then run toward the stone gates that guard the entrance to the bird sanctuary. Up I'd go on a sandy, uneven path to the large stone that marked the top. Then it was down, up, down, and then up again. I'd follow the white lines, pushing my spikes into the dirt and then listening to them clatter every time I crossed the asphalt. Eventually, I'd be back out on the open lawn, sprinting for the finish line, always near the front. My classmates on the football team were getting noticeably stronger: their biceps grew, and their shoulders broadened. I could sense the same process happening to me but on the inside. They were gaining mass and I was gaining something closer to lightness. My resting heart rate was slowing down, and my lungs had found a new rhythm. When I'd run in the woods with my teammates, we'd start to climb a hill and I'd hear their breath begin to get raspy and frequent. I'd pay attention to mine, measured and slow, like waves silently riding far up a beach and then retreating. And if the workout called for it, I'd inhale deeply and gallop off ahead.

I learned the drills, learned how to race, and learned the basic principles of getting ready: a warm body moves like water and a cold body moves like ice. Warm muscles are less likely to strain or tear than cold ones. Your hamstrings are like spaghetti: if you don't warm up, they'll be sticks, but if you stretch them too much, they'll be mush. My coach directed me toward a routine, and I dutifully followed it: I would jog, stretch, jog again, run short sprints, rest a bit, and then huddle up at the starting line. Sometimes I'd fixate on motivational phrases, including an exchange between a coach and his runner from the movie *Gallipoli*, which was about messengers in World War I.

"What are your legs?"

"Springs. Steel springs."

"What are they going to do?"

"Hurl me down the track."

"How fast can you run?"

"As fast as a leopard."

"How fast *will* you run?"

"As fast as a leopard!"

"Then let's see you do it!"

I assumed that more was better. To strengthen my core, I once did sit-ups for all three hours of *Dances with Wolves*. After losing one particularly tough race, I ran sprints up and down a hilly road by my dormitory until twilight on a rainy day. Convinced, erroneously, that a proper diet consisted of only carbohydrates—marathoners "carbo-loaded" didn't they?—I would eat four bagels and nothing else at breakfast.

Running, I began to learn, can pull you both inward and outward. When I ran, I could think more deeply than when I sat still. Whenever I broke up with a girl, I'd go run; whenever I needed an idea for a paper, I'd go run. But the sport also brought me out into the world. I would run to ponds to jump into them. If it started to pour, I would head out on the trails and take pride in the mud that splashed up until it covered my legs. I was starting to love what it felt like to move quickly among the forests as our ancestors had once done.

For some people, an obsession with running closes other doors in the mind, but it just seemed to make my internal engine run hotter: I wanted to study harder than anyone else on campus, and I wanted to run faster than anyone else in New England. I would routinely stay up most of the night working, and I'd start doing homework the minute my alarm chimed on Sunday mornings. I set up a NordicTrack cross-country skiing simulator in my dorm room and spent hours cross-training while listening to instructional cassettes about guitar playing. I look back and see a kid who was driving himself too hard. But teenage years can be treacherous if you don't have a purpose, and I had found mine. I'm proud to know that kid was me.

The summer before my senior year, I worked as an instructor at a tennis camp in the White Mountains of New Hampshire. I spent my breaks running the trails around the camp. There was one particular route I loved. I'd head up from the wooden cabins on the hill, scamper through the white pines, and then traverse the narrow, rocky trail all the way up to a fork in the road where I would turn right and head to a nearby lookout named Bald Knob. The run up took about twenty minutes, and it was a special place for me. It was on the summit that I had first kissed a girl, Carrie Politz, who had brown eyes, a lovely round face, and long, dark curly hair like a Botticelli.

After a few times running up to Bald Knob, I decided to see what would happen if I turned left at the fork and instead followed the signs to the summit of Kinsman Mountain, which was another two miles uphill. That doesn't seem far, at least until you're jumping over little streams and bounding over rocks on a path that isn't really a path. The first time I tried it, I made it about 15 minutes before my legs started to give out. I couldn't tell how far I was from the top, but I knew I wasn't close. I worried about getting lost or breaking an ankle, so I turned around. The next time, I got a little farther and a little closer to the tree line. Finally, on my third attempt, I reached a little clearing at the top. There was a light drizzle, and I couldn't see much, but I had made it to the summit. I took a deep breath of cool, windy air full of the scent of pine. I let out a little yell of exultation and then ran back down as fast as I could. A couple of days later, I took a different path and ran up Cannon Mountain. Then I went to see my family in Maine and wore out the trails up Sargent Mountain and over Penobscot. Distances and summits had ceased to be things that scared me off; they were now things that pulled me in. I wanted to go farther, higher, faster. I wanted to spend as much time as possible running above the tree line.

■

In September, I returned to Andover for my senior year and finished first, or close to it, in every race. In outdoor track, my first loss came late in the season at Northfield Mount Hermon (NMH), which was legendary for its runners, including the 1972 Olympic marathon gold medalist Frank Shorter. I had pulled a near all-nighter working on a history paper, and I drifted asleep on the bus to the campus. During the race, I was running side by side with NMH's best runner, Jason German, until, with 300 meters to go, he looked over his shoulder, glared, and said, "See you later." He then accelerated. I tried to stay with him, but my legs were just tubes of lead hanging off my hips. I finished the race, lamely muttering that he should have been disqualified for being unsportsmanlike. I remember sitting slumped in the bus, feeling like my clothes didn't fit and the flowers I had painted on my shoes were dumb. I stared at my hands, wondering why the veins were so ugly and the knuckles so large.

At this point, my warm-up routine involved stretching while listening to a specific playlist, ending with "Achilles Last Stand" by Led Zeppelin. Now, whenever I hear that song, with John Bonham furiously hammering the drums, I'm transported to the outdoor track at Deerfield Academy in western Massachusetts, where I'm getting ready for the final individual race of the New England championships. It was my chance for a rematch against German in the 3000 meters and, more important, our last chance to catch NMH for the team title. I had trained like a maniac in the weeks after my embarrassing loss, and we were far and away the two best track teams in our New England league. We had a sprinter who could run 400 meters in 47 seconds and who would later compete for the Jamaican national team; we had a shot-putter who set new records almost every weekend and who would get drafted by the Buffalo Sabres. I imagined my legs pushing into the ground at the driving rhythm of Bonham's snare drum. Then it was time to go. I put my Walkman away, steadied my breathing, and jogged to the starting line.

When runners enter the sport, it doesn't take long for them to find their race. Every person has some ratio of fast-twitch muscle fibers that help in sprints and slow-twitch muscle fibers that help at distance. Take two runners who are equal in the 1500 meters, and the one with a higher percentage of fast-twitch muscles would likely win every race that's shorter; the other would likely win every race that's longer. German was built differently from me: he was equally tall, with much more defined muscles from his legs to his arms. He had finished high school in Texas and then come north to do a postgraduate year before entering the Naval Academy. His hair was cropped short. I had hair down to my shoulders. We looked like a sixties anti-war protester and the cop about to arrest him. German would surely win a sprint, which meant I had a pretty good chance to win at the distance, which was the longest race of the day.

The gun went off and I went to the lead. My strategy was obvious: run hard, even laps of about 71 seconds each and wear German out. But maybe a lap or two in, he pulled ahead of me. Seeing him out in front again depressed me. He was better; he'd proven it earlier in the year. I sank inward and started running 72, 73, 74 seconds a lap. With two laps to go, he had about 30 meters on me. Everyone, including me, thought it was done. My teammates on the sidelines looked downcast.

Then something inside me changed. I don't know what it was or where it came from, but it's a feeling I've often tried to summon since. I suddenly felt calmer and stronger; everything inside me quieted and then intensified. I began to move faster, effortlessly. It was as though the track was now pointing down at a 10-degree angle. I started to accelerate. He was a zebra in the distance, and I was a cheetah sprinting toward him. I can still see, and feel, that gap shrinking. I almost didn't believe it.

As we went around the turn into the homestretch, with 500 meters to go, I was close. My friend Trevor Bayliss yelled the inspirational code words that we had agreed upon before the race: one was "Kinsman!" and the other was the name of my ex-girlfriend's new boyfriend. The bell clanged to signal the final lap, and I pulled even with German. Then I moved into the second lane, "the lane of high hopes," and passed him. The next minute or so was a furnace of intensity, agony, elation. I took the lead, he took it back, we pulled even, I moved ahead and into lane one. Everyone was screaming and I was sprinting. My legs hurt; my arms hurt; my vision narrowed. With 100 meters to go, I had it. Then he pulled into lane two, just off my right shoulder. We were even, and then he was ahead. I still thought I'd catch him. I had once before, hadn't I? I pushed as hard as I could.

One of the beautiful things about running is the purity of intensity it allows. I was 17 years old, and I wanted a lot of things. But this was the only one that allowed me to express that longing in its rawest form. If you want a good grade, you study hard and focus in the classroom. If you want to impress a girl, you do whatever it is that you do. If you want to make beautiful music, you practice and practice under a tree, and then you close your eyes. You don't, however, sprint and silently scream. You don't get to unleash a kind of animal anger that signals to yourself and to the world that, yes, yes, you do really want this thing. In almost everything else in life, desire is mediated by restraint. On a track, with 50 meters to go, you get to narrow your eyes and target every cell in your body toward the white line painted on the ground ahead. Your body is shaking, and your balance is no longer set. But you can go for it. This thing right here, right now.

I surged forward, my legs and arms a swirl around my blue singlet. I was just off his shoulder when I collapsed at the finish, and everything went black. When I opened my eyes, I was told that I'd come in second. I'd lost the sprint, which meant I'd lost the race, which meant our team would lose the meet. I stood up, exhausted, frustrated, and proud. Tears mixed in with my sweat. My teammates told me to keep my head up. My coach told me it was the best effort he had ever seen. I gave an interview to the school newspaper where I proclaimed, "It's the first time I haven't been upset after losing, because I know I couldn't have gone any faster."

■

I graduated from high school a few weeks later. It was raining that day, so the lunch and ceremony were held at the indoor track. My father had started drinking early that morning, trying to steel himself for the stress of seeing his former in-laws. He showed up at our table and spent hours explaining all the flaws in my mother's side of the family to the Korean immigrant parents of my closest friend and roommate. They weren't quite sure why this man was telling them so much. He added in a few of his own theories about how class works in Korea, while also mentioning all the times that he had visited dignitaries in Seoul. Both my sisters were so offended by him that they stopped eating. Afterward, he would declare to one of his friends, "I think I succeeded in demonstrating sufficient contempt toward my ex-wife without being rude." My mother, meanwhile, paid as little attention as possible to her ex. She went about her business making new friends and catching up with old ones. He wanted to get under her skin. She wanted to ignore him. "You despise me, don't you?" asks Ugarte, in my father's favorite movie, *Casablanca*. "If I gave you any thought, I probably would," responds Rick.

The last award to be announced was the Aurelian Honor Society Award, which was determined by faculty nominations and student votes. When my name was called, my father lost control and jumped out of his seat. He charged through the other parents, knocking over empty white plastic chairs, and bolted up to the stage to give me a big hug. He wrote in his memoir, "When it was announced that the winner was Nicholas Edwin Scott Thompson, I literally lost it. I surely climbed over the shoulders and laps of 500 people to get to the stage and give my son a congratulatory hug before anyone else got there."

I probably should have been mortified. My drunken father had crashed the stage and shifted the spotlight from me to him. But all I remember is being slightly amused. Like him, I had started as a lonely outsider at this school. Like him, I had learned how to work hard and to catch up. Unlike him, I had learned to be at ease with my peers. I had become, in many ways, the student that my father had wanted to be, and he was thrilled.

CHAPTER 3

Bobbi Gibb

You put one foot in front of the other, and you breathe this air. I can't get over it. I can't get over the fact that it all exists.

—BOBBI GIBB

AS MY FATHER PLOWED THROUGH THE CHAIRS THAT DAY AT ANDOVER, there was another woman in the audience who would come to mean a lot to me. Her name was Bobbi Gibb and she was watching her son graduate. He was a friend of mine, but I didn't know him well enough to realize that his mother, out on one of the plastic chairs on the track, was maybe the most important runner ever to visit the school. In time, I would learn that she had the purest idea of the sport of anyone I've ever known.

Bobbi Gibb was born in 1942, the same year as my father. She grew up in suburban Boston and had the childhood of a fox cub. She roamed the woods around her home, exploring. Her parents weren't quite sure what to do with her. Her father was a chemistry professor and her mother lived what Gibb considered the deadening life of a housewife, popping tranquilizers and trying to smile obediently when her husband came home. "How are you going to find a husband, running in the woods?" Gibb's mother asked her.

In the spring of 1964, when she was 21, her father took her to watch the Boston Marathon. She had no concept of the race. She didn't know how many miles it was or why anyone did it. But, as she and her father stood on the side, near the midpoint of the course, she saw a miracle in the runners. They looked so balanced; their footsteps were almost silent. She felt a kinship and a connection. "It was just people running: strong and quiet. Something that was so human," she told me. When she and I met, she was 79, but she remembered everything about those runners. She told me that she felt she had found her people. It was, she says, "like falling in love." She didn't even register that everybody on the road was a man.

Gibb wanted to do it herself, and that summer she decided to train by traveling. She had saved a few hundred dollars working as a camp counselor, and her parents were in Europe for the summer. So she just hopped into her family's pale-yellow VW microbus and headed west. She traveled by back roads with only her dog, a malamute named Moot, as company. She'd find a forest, park the van, and run for hours. If she got lost, Moot would help her find her way back. Gibb was like Artemis, who ran through the woods with her hunting dogs. She and Moot would sleep outside under the trees, with Gibb wrapped in an Indian blanket. She would let the amphibians sing her to sleep. They started in the Berkshires, then headed to the farm country of New York State. She was looking for quiet places or the spots "between the names." She brought binoculars to examine the stars at night.

She passed through West Virginia and through Ohio. She visited relatives in Indiana and slept in their backyard. She stopped at a farm in Kansas where a woman lived with her paralyzed son. Her husband had left her because she would not institutionalize the child. Gibb stayed for a few days and earned money by painting the woman's fences. She ran in the Great Plains. She ran in the Rockies and slept in a field of wildflowers. One morning, while running, she jumped over a bush and nearly landed in a mineshaft. She stayed with a friend in a trailer camp in Wyoming and marveled at the sky above the Nevada desert. But mostly she was on her own: running, running, running. She didn't log her runs, and she doesn't remember exactly where she went. She didn't even own a watch. She would just park, set up camp, and then look for mountaintops in the distance and head toward them. One day, out west, a group of horses formed a circle around her, noses in. She spoke gently with them, and soon they started running with her.

She was running to be free and to be spiritually connected to the earth. She was also running away from a society designed by and for men. "Women were so restricted," she told me. "You couldn't have a credit card, you couldn't be a doctor, couldn't be a lawyer. If you were a woman you had to be in this little box. You had to get married. It was like *Pride and Prejudice*. I grew up fuming about this. It was thought improper for a grown woman to run in public. And there I am running with horses."

The journey ended when she plunged into the churning waves of the Pacific Ocean, just north of San Francisco on Stinson Beach. "Running is a fantastic way to be outdoors," she said to me. "You put one foot in front of the other, and you breathe this air. I can't get over it. I can't get over the fact that it all exists." The sport, she told me, "is the way that I feel at one with the universe."

■

In the fall of 1965, Gibb decided to try a 100-mile horse race in the Green Mountains of Vermont. Gibb figured she could just slip herself in. The horses and their riders started out one at a time in the center of town, and Gibb trotted out among them at dawn. The miles were marked with different-colored circles, which meant this was one of the first times Gibb knew how far she was running. Most of the time she was alone, but occasionally she'd pass a horse, or a horse would pass her. "Are you going the whole way?" a rider would ask. "I hope so," she'd respond. The first day, she drank at the horse troughs and didn't eat anything. She covered 40 miles and was offered a carrot by a spectator when she finished.

The next day, Gibb covered another 25 miles. Her knees had started to ache, but she had accomplished her goal: convincing herself that she could run the Boston Marathon the following spring. She hitchhiked to a nearby town and took a bus home.

She had started to date a boy who was a student at Harvard. One day, he had to make a quick stop at Lamont Library on campus. Gibb went in with him, but the attendant stopped her and declared, "No women allowed in the library." Gibb lost it. "Me? Not allowed in a *library* because I'm a woman?" She let out a series of primal screams until the words came to her. "What do you think a woman is going to do in your precious library . . . read? Maybe think? Maybe . . . contribute something to society, perhaps . . . learn something? Discover something?"

She turned and sprinted out the door. She ran down to the Charles River and then turned right and followed its path, racing the men in a crew boat as they rowed. She traveled the winding path all the way up to Watertown, five miles west, before finally turning around and heading back to Cambridge.

A few months later, she sent a letter to the organizers of the Boston Marathon requesting an application form for entry. They wrote back and said, no. Women, the organizers declared, are not physically capable of running marathons, and the organizers did not want to take on the liability risk. Gibb considered this absurd. She had been keeping pace with horses; why would she have any problem with men?

Evolution has given men some physiological advantages over women while running. Men have more testosterone and higher oxygen-uptake capacities. They generally have less fat and bigger muscles. Women's bodies have different angles, which makes it harder for them to generate explosive power. Breasts have complicated physics that can disrupt forward motion, particularly if not in a well-fitting sports bra. But women's bodies are designed to do something more painful, and consequential, than a marathon: give birth. Because of this, women are better at preserving carbohydrates, and they store extra fats, which can be helpful over long races. Research also shows that they tend to be smarter about pacing and are more likely to run even splits. As my Andover contemporary Christine Yu noted in her wonderful book, *Up to Speed: The Groundbreaking Science of Women Athletes*, men do about 10 percent better than women in short races and marathons. When the race gets to 50 miles, men do about 4 percent better. Once the race gets to 200 miles or longer, women perform slightly better.

Gibb crumpled up the letter from the Boston Athletic Association, threw it on the floor, and then ran 20 miles to Del Mar Beach, near San Diego, where she had moved. She slept out on the sand and woke up to the sound of waves and the realization that now she had even more reason to run the race. "Suddenly," she told me, "my running took on a meaning greater than my own enjoyment." When April came, Gibb took a bus east across the country and headed to her parents' house.

For years, Gibb's mother, Jean, had scolded Gibb and tried to squeeze her into conformity and domesticity. The morning of the race, though, Jean switched teams. Gibb's father stormed out of the house when he learned that his daughter was going to break the rules and run the Boston Marathon. Jean decided to drive Gibb to the start, covering the course in reverse so Gibb would get a sense of it. Jean said she was proud of her daughter. "Mom, you're on my side for the first time," Gibb said. "It's something I should have done a long time ago," Jean replied. She apologized that she had spent so many years trying to crush the young woman's spirit. "Thank God I failed," Jean said.

Joan of Arc dressed as a man to fight in the Hundred Years' War. Charlotte Brontë published her novels under the name Currer Bell. And now there was Bobbi Gibb, hiding in the yellow forsythia bush near the race's start in borrowed shorts, a bathing suit, and a sweatshirt, with the hood up over her head. She waited for the gun, sneaked her way into the middle of a pack of runners, and took off at a sub-seven-minutes-per-mile pace.

The disguise didn't work very well. Shortly into the race, one of the men behind Gibb hollered out that he thought there was a girl ahead of him. Soon the whole group of men she was with realized that they had a woman in their midst. Pioneers who break gender or racial barriers aren't always welcomed, but Gibb was. The men knew it was against the rules, but they loved it. Gibb said she was overheating and wanted to take off her sweatshirt. "It's a free road," one of the men said.

Word started to spread that a woman was running. The news traveled from the road to the local radio stations and then to the fans up ahead. As Gibb passed Wellesley College—where my mother was a freshman along with Hillary Rodham—women stood by the side screaming. "Do it, girl! Go! Go! Go! Go!" Gibb saw a woman with several children holding on to her large overcoat. Tears were streaming down her cheeks as she shouted, "Ave Maria."

Gibb held on to her pace to the start of the Newton Hills. But she hadn't drunk any water and her feet were blistering. She took off her shoes and tried to go barefoot. That hurt too much, so she put the shoes back on and hobbled along. She finished in three hours and twenty-one minutes.

Soon after she crossed the line, the governor of Massachusetts came up to shake her hand. Afterward, she took a taxi back to her parents' house and saw cars parked up and down the street. She thought one of her neighbors must be having a party and was startled to learn from her parents that the press had shown up. The next day's *Boston Globe* ran the headline, "Girl Finishes Marathon."

Bobbi Gibb ran the 1967 Boston Marathon too. This time, she stayed out of the forsythia bushes and headed out proudly with the rest of the runners, wearing an ornate patterned jacket but no race number. She hadn't registered for the race because she knew she wouldn't get in. The Boston Marathon was classified as a "men's division race," which meant women simply weren't allowed. If a woman formally finished, all the men's times could be invalidated. Gibb ran in 1968 too. But that was enough. She had proven her point.

I spent a lot of time talking with Gibb over the course of several years, trying to understand the source of her courage that day in 1966. She wanted to prove that women could do something most people thought they couldn't. She wanted to accomplish something for herself: "That was the first goal that I had decided I was going to do. It was something that I was meant to do," she told me. But, even more, she did it out of love for the sport, for the ground, and for the open air: "When you're running, you don't have to think about what your boss wants you to do that day. You're free. You feel the energy of the universe blowing through you."

Gibb now lives in eastern Massachusetts. She's in her early 80s and she doesn't run much out on the roads, but she still spends an hour or so a day running on a small indoor trampoline facing the woods. We met in a coffee shop with wide views of the beach and then she showed me her home, which is roughly 98-percent artist's studio and 2-percent living space. Her memory of the first race is vivid from having told the story so many times, but she had run other marathons in the years since. When I asked her for her fastest finishing time, she couldn't quite figure it out. Finally, she said, it was in the 1980s in New York, but she wasn't sure what year. I looked it up and there it was: 3:19 in the 1982 New York City Marathon. She had finished not long after my father the year he had run his best time. I told her that I must have seen her go by, standing just past the Queensboro Bridge, where I had given my father a new pair of shoes. She looked at me and said, "I hope I touched your hand."

CHAPTER 4

Just Thanks

The only advantage for a child in having an alcoholic parent is that you acquire, prematurely, quite a bit of valuable data.

—GORE VIDAL

MY FATHER'S ACADEMIC SUCCESS AT ANDOVER WON HIM A SCHOLARship to Stanford, where he thrived like no other time in his life. His classmates remember him as a flurry of energy, wit, and charisma. Even now, there's a kind of love and awe in their memories. He was elected to run the Political Union and the Institute of International Relations. He organized a coup by which he and other ambitious students took over a moribund fraternity, changing it from a site of bacchanalian revelry to one of Ciceronian debate. He was featured constantly in *The Stanford Daily*. The *Stanford Review* ran an article about him called "The College Student" and noted, "Yes, that's another picture of Scotty Thompson. Yes, this is something of a Thompson issue." He brought Barry Goldwater, Richard Nixon, and John F.

Kennedy to campus. When Kennedy arrived, my father drove a limousine to San Francisco to pick him up. As my father would recount the story, he was greeted by the then-senator, who was wearing a terrycloth robe, in his penthouse room at a hotel near the airport. Kennedy introduced my father to a woman named Judith Campbell, later Exner, who was most certainly not the senator's wife. The two men drove to Stanford, where they were stopped by a security guard near Memorial Auditorium, which was mobbed. "What the hell are you doing? Don't you realize Senator Kennedy is coming?" the guard asked. My father reached back and unrolled the window. "Oh my God," the security guard said.

The Saturday Evening Post ran a story about my father in which Kennedy was quoted saying that Scotty Thompson might make it to the White House before he did. A Stanford classmate also quoted in the article said, "I'm sick and tired of listening to the bull sessions on 'Is there a God?' and 'What makes Scotty Thompson tick?'" One faculty member later recounted a story in which my father was washing dishes in a dormitory, took off his apron, and went to borrow the president of the school's limousine to go pick up Vice President Richard Nixon at the airport.

His obsession in his senior year was winning a Rhodes Scholarship, the pinnacle of collegiate academic and social achievement in that era. Decades later, I wrote to the Rhodes Trust and was sent the recommendation letters that the Stanford faculty had written. They did not disappoint. "Scotty Thompson is the kind of young man that comes along only once in approximately ten years," wrote the Stanford dean of students. "I cannot recall ever having known a student who possessed the same combination of intelligence, creativity, energy, drive, and dedication." "He has attempted more, and achieved more, than anyone we have studied—including some who now hold high office," wrote the director of the Alumni Association. "He is generally conceded among those who have observed the student body since World War II to be the outstanding student leader of the era," wrote James T. Watkins, the director of the International Relations Program in a letter that went on for six pages. "I think it likely that, in the entire history of Stanford campus life, he has had no near rival since Herbert Hoover was an undergraduate."

My father won the Rhodes, which gave him a scholarship to Oxford and an entry pass into a world of poetry, Greek vases, and High Table dinners. As his star rose, it eclipsed that of his own father, who had become inseparable from his gin bottle. Men often struggle when they start to feel that they don't matter as much as they did before. Frank had asked my father to convince the president of Stanford to get him a job at another school in the University of California system. The request embarrassed my father, who explained why this wasn't possible. He was now ahead in a competition with his father that he had hated losing but that he dearly wanted not to win. In a diary entry a decade later, my father wrote, "I associate my gains with his losses (and so does he, I think)."

After completing his first year at Oxford, my father began traveling throughout Africa. On one trip, he shared a room with a grandson of King George V, Prince William of Gloucester. One night, in Ghana, in 1966, my father heard guns blasting at two in the morning and an announcement over the radio that the government of Kwame Nkrumah had fallen. Naturally, he headed over to the presidential palace, where papers were being thrown into fires. My father ran into the mayhem and emerged with all the documents he could carry. He brought them back on a motorbike to his bungalow. A month later, he was arrested and briefly put in jail for mysterious reasons. He was soon released, likely, he noted, with some nudging from the CIA. My father used the documents as the basis for his dissertation and then to help him write an article for *The Atlantic Monthly*, in which he argued that the West had an obligation to help nurture democracies in the newly independent states of Africa. Getting published in such a prestigious magazine gave my father further confidence. It was a feat that "seemed to keep my fire, of future success, burning back home."

■

My father's most important connection at Oxford turned out to be Bill Nitze, the bookish son of Paul Nitze, then the secretary of the Navy and soon the undersecretary of defense. After my father returned to the United States with a DPhil, Bill introduced him to his sister, Nina Nitze, a beautiful, sophisticated, and brilliant undergraduate at Wellesley. She was the youngest of four children and had grown up in a household where people such as Walter Lippmann, Dean Acheson, and George Kennan would stop by for dinner. Her paternal grandfather was an eminent scholar of Arthurian literature. Her maternal grandmother had been the first female congresswoman from New York. Her mother was one of the most respected, and sometimes feared, women in Washington. My mother combined the best traits from all these lines. She was wickedly smart and cultured. She also had, my father would later tell me, the most beautiful voice he had ever heard.

She fell immediately for the quick-witted, ambitious Rhodes

Scholar. They were soon engaged, and my father fully entered the life and wealthier world he had imagined while hiding behind the curtains in his Oklahoma home. For decades, I've had a photograph on top of my dressing bureau of my mother dancing with her father at the wedding. She's wearing a gorgeous full-length veil that had been passed down for generations. She looks impossibly young, as all parents do to their children in wedding photos. My grandfather's collar is up and he has a carnation pinned to his lapel. He's smiling. It was the last month of the Johnson Administration. He was 61 years old, and he had another twenty years of high-level government service to go.

This world thrilled my father. Still, at times he felt like a trespasser. After Oxford, he knew how to attach cuff links and how to use a salad fork. But he couldn't play tennis; he talked too much about money. (He never quite caught on to the rule of the East Coast establishment that you're supposed to get and protect as much money as you can, but that speaking of it is considered vulgar.) He once stood in a swimming pool denouncing Britain's actions during the 1956 Suez Canal crisis without realizing that he was talking to the former foreign secretary who had guided the country during the crisis. When I was a child, he tried to teach his in-laws, who had been skiing in Aspen for decades, a lesson in efficiency and put our skis, with the boots attached, on the roof of his car overnight. Everything froze solid and we couldn't get our feet in them the next morning.

My father continued to move fast during the early years of his marriage. He began publishing books; he made plans to run for office and persuaded my mother to buy a farm in New Hampshire, partly because he thought he might find a path to the Senate in the "Live Free or Die" state. His politics shifted rightward and began to more closely match his father-in-law's.

But he also started drinking too much, smoking too much, going out too much. Many of his diary entries from the 1970s are about his struggles with alcohol. Three weeks before my birth, he wrote: "A smoker is aware of his hack; a drinker enjoys the soporific or stupefying effect and his drinking dulls the consciousness of the depth of the problem, at least until the next day. And then when the evening comes, one can always say, just one: which makes #2 so much easier, to say nothing of what #2 does for #3."

I was born, quite prematurely, in the summer of 1975. Here, my father's diary stops. He couldn't handle the possibility that I might not survive. I spent weeks in an incubator, with my exhausted mother sitting by my side, poking one finger in through a hole in the Plexiglas. My body became so hot that I was placed on a bed of ice, but my father didn't visit. She was giving me life; he was terrified of death. It was a betrayal of me that would later haunt him. When my dad's diary resumes, he notes that the worst of my medical crisis was over and that he was still trying to sort out his own. "One starts with life expanding—rather I started—with life expanding more or less continuously until my twenties.... Then it all began narrowing down as the reality of my lack of control and the reality of my inability to fulfil my needs and ambitions.... And all could be solved relatively rapidly if I could stop drinking."

It was around this time that my father started to jog. Drinking and running are mirror opposites. One makes you feel great while you do it and dismal afterward; the other does the reverse. Completing a run can give you an excuse to take a drink or a reason to abstain. To my father, at least at this point, the goal was to try to find something that could bring discipline into the alcohol-pickled mayhem of his days. Running also masked athletic weakness, as he would later tell me, because running was the rare sport where you mostly competed against yourself. You could learn without having to lose.

Initially, my father just ran two or three miles a day. The first reference in his diaries comes shortly after I came home from the hospital. "I am back on track, with calisthenics building up and jogging really on." A few months later, his young son kept him up at night, but he felt better: "I am in fine shape: I jogged three miles this afternoon, down to Memorial Bridge."

By the late 1970s, my father's inner life was unraveling but his professional life was finally coming together. He would get up at 6 A.M. and, if in Boston, play *Star Wars* figures with me in his office down in the basement. He'd then go for a run and head off to work. He was earning a name as a young public intellectual making the hawkish case for prosecuting the Cold War. He won a White House Fellowship and earned tenure. He traveled around the country for television appearances and debates, including, most unfortunately, one at the Heritage Foundation on the long-scheduled day that my little sister, Heidi, was born by cesarean section. In one memorable exchange, he was debating arms control. His interlocutor declared that my father stood only for the Republican Party but that she stood for all of humanity. "That may be true," my father responded, "but at least I was appointed to my position."

When Ronald Reagan was elected president, my father became a candidate for top foreign-policy jobs in the new administration. One day many decades later, I came upon the document ranking Reagan's team's picks for every key role. My father's name is typed next to the number 1 to run the State Department's Policy Planning staff, along with a note: "Dr. Scott Thompson: Fletcher; good commendations." Above it, handwritten is another "1" and the name "Paul Wolfowitz." My father ended up in a good job several levels down the bureaucracy. Wolfowitz got the position running Policy Planning, and then many bigger ones in the years to come. My father never knew how close he had come.

Meanwhile, my father was losing control of his repressed sexual feelings toward men. In his memoir, he describes a link between his homosexual awakening and his professional success. "There was now only the slightest gap between the cup of my life and the lip of political fulfillment I had spent my life seeking. I was quickly to discern that it is always at that point that the impulse to slip—indeed to throw it away—is greatest; perhaps if only because for some, life's purpose lies essentially only in the awakening quest—and to show that you can do without what you have worked so hard for."

His life, both career and family, was working in the ways he had envisioned since childhood, but he was about to detonate it all because of a relationship with a 25-year-old chemical engineer at MIT named Mark Altbush. There was one last party—a glamorous 40th-birthday celebration for my father with gold-and-black balloons and 90 guests—and then he was gone, off to Washington. The basement office was emptied. I spent hours upon hours there, practicing floor hockey by myself.

It was in this period of self-destruction and self-realization that running became part of my father's identity. He knew he needed a new life. He started eating better and training more. He would squeeze in runs at 5 A.M., heading out in a headband and colored shorts that were maybe a bit too short. After he ran the New York City Marathon in 1982, he drove back to Washington. He showed up in front of a class he was teaching at Georgetown in his shiny silver finisher's blanket, as though he had just run the race. He told the class that it was the only thing that he had in the car to help shield him from the rain, and then he mentioned how fast his time had been. Tracy Bennett, one of his female graduate students, told me years later, "He was flamboyant, gently endearing, annoyingly arrogant, piercingly intelligent, entertaining, and more. I'd never met a man—nor had a professor—who was clearly so brilliant and at the same time so precariously insecure."

Bennett, who began a short relationship with him, believed running was a centripetal force that held my father's life together. "Running was a way that he built discipline that translated to the rest of his life. When he was running, he was drinking less, and he was focused on his work. He used the time to process everything that was going on in his head," she said.

The relationship didn't last long. His running slowed and his drinking accelerated. Bennett would sometimes have to drive him home from work after lunch so he could sleep off his libations. Or she'd just tuck him in on the office couch and hope no one important came by. They broke up not long after she discovered a letter he had written to a male graduate student, so full of tenderness and affection that she knew he must be gay. My father once told me that one has the ability to resist the first affair in a relationship, but once the dam is broken, the waters flood out. The difference from zero to one affair is large; the difference between one and a hundred, he explained, is small.

Soon after the end of his relationship with Bennett, my father received the most traumatic news of his life. He visited a doctor in Washington who pronounced that he was HIV positive. "In a sense, I felt liberated," he later wrote. "The fit outcome of this interminable ordeal was to be not redemption but death."

I was 10 years old when he told me that he was going to be dead within a year and that he wanted me to be OK without him. We were in the car, just the two of us, on Interstate 66 in Virginia. I was sitting in the passenger seat, and I didn't quite understand. I tried to laugh and tell him that yes, I knew everyone died, but he wasn't going to. But he was sincere. He didn't want to go into the details, but he really needed me to listen. He wanted me to know that he loved me, and that I would be OK without him. I bottled the news deep inside. I never told anyone else.

A year later, he enrolled in a study on healthy HIV-positive men. Shortly thereafter, he got a call from Anthony Fauci, then the director of the National Institute of Allergy and Infectious Diseases, calmly saying that he would be removed from the study because he didn't have the disease after all. "We ran the test three ways," Fauci declared in a crisp, no-nonsense voice. My father walked outside into the spring sunshine, elated and unsettled. A few weeks later he told me that, actually, he was going to be fine. In later years, he would say that Fauci had "sentenced me to life."

I still didn't know for sure that he was gay, and it wasn't until I was 13 that he told me. We were staying with his sister, my Aunt Sue, at her home in Los Angeles, but my father and I had driven down to San Diego to visit SeaWorld in the morning. Afterward, we had gone to a movie theater to see *Dead Poets Society*. As we drove back north, my father tried to explain his sexuality. He told me that the man who lived in his house, Jack, was gay, but that he hadn't known it when they'd met. When he found out, he told me, as I wrote in my diary that evening, "the only thing that bothered him was that Jack dated and pretended to love women. He also said that he and Jack were 'affectionate friends.'" He asked me if I wanted to ask him any questions. I said I did not.

I wish I had been more inquisitive then. I had never met anyone who I knew was gay, and because this was 1988, I'd never even seen a gay character on the screen. My only understanding was from a classmate's mother, who had once pointed out the window, while we drove to school, at a man who walked in an effeminate way and wore a colorful jacket. "That's a homosexual," she declared.

So that guy was a homosexual, and now, so was Jack and so probably was my father. I could have asked a thousand things. But emotional curiosity wasn't my strength as a child, and my father did not excel at this kind of parenting conversation. We kept driving back to Los Angeles. Later, we went for a jog together and talked about something else.

■

The summer after my graduation from high school, I received a letter from Vin Lananna, the new cross-country coach at Stanford, where I was enrolled for the fall. It came in a white envelope with a single stamp, and it slammed me right in the gut.

The letter gave us instructions for getting ready for the season: We were to run about fifty miles a week at about seven minutes a mile. We had some workouts to do, and every now and then he wanted us to find golf courses where we could sprint from one hole to another and do push-ups or sit-ups on the green. Then it detailed the terrifying exploits of the most promising boys in the incoming freshman class. Lananna had successfully recruited the second-, third-, and seventh-place finishers from the national high school cross-country championships. Besides those three, there were six other recruits faster than I was, most of whom had been state champions. My name was listed without a bio. The letter added that runners should ideally weigh two pounds for every inch of height. That sounded fine until I did the math: I was 6'1" and weighed 165. That made me 19 pounds overweight. This was the era in which Mark Wetmore, the legendary coach of the University of Colorado Buffaloes, said, "Go look at *Track & Field News*. See what those people look like. You should look like a skeleton with a condom pulled over your skull."

I was 18 years old, a Roman candle of emotions, ambitions, and hormones. I wanted to out-run and out-train all those state champions. In high school, I had run roughly 35 miles every week; now I did 70. I would often bike 20 miles out to Walden Pond and then run in Thoreau's woods. I ran a race in Cambridge where I stayed right on the shoulder of Lynn Jennings, who had won a bronze medal at 10,000 meters in the Barcelona Olympics the summer before. I kept a book called *The Warrior Athlete* close at hand. I read Arthur Schlesinger's biographies of JFK and RFK on my mother's patio while doing hamstring and quad stretches nearly the entire time.

Training like that does make one faster, just as charging straight into a stuck door will often knock it open. But there's usually a better way to do it. Sure enough, the week I was to show up on campus, I felt a piercing pain in my shin while running sprints on a pine path in the Arnold Arboretum in Boston.

It was faint and awkward at first: like a bee sting. Then it felt like a shark bite. I had to stop and then limp home. A day or two later, my mother and I showed up in Palo Alto and stayed at a hotel on El Camino Real. I went to meet Lananna and told him about my shin. He sent me off on my bicycle to the Stanford medical center, where I learned that I had developed a stress fracture before my first workout with the team.

I missed the whole fall season and had to train by treading water in a running motion in the diving pool. I would shuffle quickly from the locker room, hoping no one noticed the acne on my back, and jump into the 25-yard heated pool. It was a lovely spot—young Stanford divers doing somersaults in the afternoon sunshine—if you were a swimmer. It wasn't so great if you were an injured runner sputtering around the back wall like a dog thrown off a boat. I passed the time by playing "questions" from the Tom Stoppard play *Rosencrantz and Guildenstern Are Dead* with another hobbled teammate. "Do you want to start?" "Are you asking me?" "Who else would I be talking to?" In early November, I was ready to run a single mile on the soft grass of the football field. It felt great to be a land mammal again. The next day, I was diagnosed with mononucleosis.

I eventually was able to run with the team, but it's hard to catch up when you start in last place and then miss several months. I was a Toyota racing Ferraris and my tires were flat. I remember running alone up the wide paths of the Stanford foothills as my teammates descended out of sight. I lived three doors down from the top recruit on the women's cross-country team, a Teutonic goddess who was the daughter of an All-Pro NFL linebacker. When teammates said they wanted to come by my dorm and say hello to me, I generally assumed they wanted an excuse to ask her to dinner. One day, in the dorm's dining room, I complained that I was tired because of how hard I had trained. She happened to hear and added, "You shouldn't be tired. I should be tired." Then she detailed her workouts, which included not just her runs for the cross-country team but her early-morning training on the swim team. She wasn't wrong. But it made me feel tiny and hopeless, like a grasshopper stuffed into a mason jar.

Coach Lananna had studied elite Kenyan distance runners and wanted his runners to do some of the things they did—and some things they didn't. He had us run strides barefoot after workouts to teach the tendons and muscles in our feet to connect to the ground. He believed that many injuries came from inefficient form and that inefficient form sometimes came from bulky shoes. He had us lift weights in the mornings. He had the runners get massages—a rare practice then and a common one now. It was very clear that he was something of a sorcerer. Our team got remarkably better every week.

One Wednesday, Lananna warned us in advance that we would have a hard workout the next day. I doodled nervously while taking notes in Thursday's Literature and the Arts class, sketching cartoon characters with overlarge pointed ears. Surely, I would be last again. My one hope was that the workout would take place in Eucalyptus Grove near the track, where you could disappear, not around the track in the giant stadium where everyone would notice long-haired Nick struggling in the back. I bicycled down to the locker room and was informed that we would be doing 12 400-meter runs with one minute rest after each one. Twelve laps around the track, in full view of everyone. But then something miraculous happened: I kept up. I stayed conservatively at the very back on the first few, then confidently moved to the middle. Afterward, I ran barefoot sprints with my teammates down the football field and then did sit-ups in the grass. For one day, I felt the golden Palo Alto sun shining down on Stanford Stadium. Maybe, just maybe, I was good enough.

Lananna's next workout for us, a few days later, was sets of 200-meter repeats. Unfortunately, I had stayed up almost the entire night before preparing for a chemistry test. I was taking the maximum number of classes and obsessed with getting straight As. This is a good way to learn. But it's not the right way to recover. During each repeat, just 50 meters in, I was off the pack. I watched the other runners gliding ahead of me. I was alone and quite literally last. Each time, I felt like a child, hopelessly reaching up as the balloon I'd been holding floated skyward.

I filled my diary with lamentations about running. I wasn't good enough and would never be. Why was I spending 20 hours a week humiliating myself? Finally, one day, late in the spring, I went for a run in the foothills above campus. I stopped, took off my shoes, and sat barefoot staring out toward San Francisco Bay. Why waste so much time running when there was so much life going on everywhere else on campus? I decided that I wasn't going to do it next year.

Quitting the team was hard, but not running was easy. In my sophomore year, I joined the environmental group and was quickly pulled into the world of campus politics. I became the student my father wanted me to be. I was eventually elected vice president of the Stanford student government and the coordinator of other national student groups. I brought political figures to campus, including several third-party presidential candidates. (One difference between father and son: Ralph Nader did not greet me in a terrycloth robe, thank god.) The campus newspaper ran a long, glowing profile of me, which I sent to my father. It quoted me saying, "It's not the end of the world for children to have gay parents," and that "living with him and the prejudice against him helped me develop a little bit of a social conscience." My father said that he was extremely proud, but he chastised me for having declared in a quote that I had grown up "upper middle-class." If Paul Nitze's grandson wasn't upper-class, who was?

I also wrote about my father's sexuality in my own column for *The Stanford Daily*. After it was published, the conservative paper on campus, *The Stanford Review*, published a short note: "Last week Nick Thompson wrote an impassioned plea for openness toward homosexuality in society. We can think of one more argument in support. If society had been more open, perhaps his father wouldn't have gotten married and then we wouldn't have to deal with Nick." I sent the clip to my father, who framed it and hung it in his living room.

It was at about this time that I asked my father whether he had ever thought I might be gay. I had never felt any attraction to men and I'd had an inexhaustible, if generally unreciprocated, attraction to the girls in my schools. Still, I was my father's son and he clearly hadn't figured it out until he was 40. No, he said, he'd known I was going to be straight since he had seen me observing a babysitter in her bathing suit when I was about 10. It was soon after that when I started to wear a pink triangle on my backpack in solidarity with the gay and lesbian students on campus.

Even as I immersed myself in politics, though, running was never completely out of mind, and I watched Lananna turn my classmates into the best runners in the country. My senior year, the team won the men's national championship, and the women's team, which he also coached, won the title too. The next year, the men won it again.

A quarter-century after I quit the team, I called Lananna. My mother has always referred to him as "the man who broke my son," but I've been more sympathetic. I broke myself by training too hard. Plus, the man knew how to win. He took a Bad News Bears team and turned it into the Yankees. Lananna had previously coached at Dartmouth, and he told me that coming to Palo Alto had made him realize just how much harder it is to train a team where the roads are iced over four months a year. But Stanford had its challenges as well. "There was so much pressure for you guys to do well in the classroom," he said. Students who came "to get this great elite academic experience" weren't going to succeed on the cross-country team. The runners who succeeded were smart kids who were content to get Bs. Athletics and academics were at odds. "As much as we liked to say they were compatible, they were not compatible," he said. It's the thing that everyone knows at Stanford but that no one is supposed to say. Lananna went on to coach at the University of Oregon. There, he added, "kids merely expected to run well and the other stuff was not going to get in the way."

I had called Lananna partly to reminisce, partly because he's one of the geniuses of the sport, and partly because I wanted a better understanding of my time on the team. When I quit, I assumed I didn't have the talent. Based on how fast I've run since, that seems wrong. Part of the problem, as I realized during the call, was that I cared about other things too much. But the main reason is more interesting. I realize now that I've sought distinct and different compound goals from the sport as I've gone through life: self-confidence, self-awareness, and self-transcendence. None is necessarily better than the others, but as I've gotten older I've learned to balance them. But back then, at age 21, it was almost all about self-confidence. I didn't understand then that you could run hard just to teach yourself new things about yourself, your goals, and what it means to be a human inside a flawed physical body. I might have kept at the sport if I had realized that you can run just to understand yourself; you don't always have to run to win.

You can't unspool just one thread from the tapestry of life, though. And if I could go back, I wouldn't change a thing. Leaving running led me to play guitar more intently. I'd practice on the porch, on the roof, in the foothills. I slept on the roof of my dorm every night, under the stars, and I'd often practice right until I drifted off, guitar by my side. I was developing my own idiosyncratic style: open tunings, drone notes, slaps, and mathematical patterns. I couldn't read music or play in a band. But I got better and better. I was developing calluses on my fingers while I cleared my mind.

Then, one day in my junior year, a stunning woman named Danielle Goldman walked into the campus coffeehouse while I was onstage playing my acoustic guitar. She had beautiful shoulder-length brown hair, and lovely light freckles under her fair blue eyes. She sat quietly at the side and must have heard something she liked because she sent a two-word email: "just thanks." I responded quickly and added her name to the mailing list to which I sent out details on upcoming concerts. A few days later, I released my first album, titled *Red Weather* after a line in my favorite poem. I sent a note to the list, and she responded, "Like the Wallace Stevens poem?" We started corresponding, and I decided she was the smartest person I'd ever met. She was a year older than I was and about to graduate and go off to study at the London Contemporary Dance School. We went for a walk early one morning around the dry Lake Lagunita and then she departed. We figured we probably wouldn't see each other in person again, which in some ways was freeing. We started writing letters. I told her all about my father. "We don't write about frivolity just because we think it's important to keep in touch," I wrote in my journal. "We have no reason to keep in touch and so we only write about what really matters." A year later, she came back to America, and we've been together since.

Even as my life began to come together, I was chased by the ambitions my father had set for me. He had told me from about age 10 that I was destined to win the Rhodes Scholarship, just like he had. In my junior year, I had won a Truman Scholarship, which seemed like a precursor to the big prize. It was not to be. After I lost, one of the judges on the interview committee wrote to me: "Your intelligence and energy came across well, but it felt as though you were very anxious to appear to have answers to every issue; it didn't feel like a conversation that moved naturally forward, a dialogue driven by questions. For myself, I will say that trite though it may sound, you don't seem to have found any inner peace with yourself."

My recollection of losing is just sadness. But digging through old emails, I found at least one note that suggested something else. Directly after finding out that I had lost, I wrote "I AM LIBERATED" in an email to Danielle. "Despite trying my damnedest, I got bounced from the Rhodes. . . . Now, I have released the monkey on my back named Expectations."

CHAPTER 5

A Tiny Imperceptible Tailwind

Only the disciplined ones in life are free. If you are undisciplined, you are a slave to your moods and your passions.
—ELIUD KIPCHOGE, TWO-TIME OLYMPIC MARATHON
GOLD MEDALIST FOR KENYA

AFTER COLLEGE, I MOVED TO NEW HAMPSHIRE TO CONCENTRATE ON playing guitar and applying for jobs. I had a notion that I could somehow combine my idiosyncratic fingerpicking with the fusion funk of John McLaughlin. I would practice eight hours a day and, through monkish dedication, extract a sound I couldn't even really hear in my head.

It didn't last long. I wasn't getting close to the sound I wanted. So, about a month into my woodshedding, sitting by a granite wall and feeling lonely, I decided to try racing for the first time in four years. I took my father's goal and made it my own: I would try to run a three-hour marathon. I registered for an upcoming race in Rhode Island and invited my father to do it with me, but he demurred. My training consisted of running a few days a week and hiking through the White Mountains on others. Meanwhile, I applied for jobs and, after several interviews, was hired for a role at *60 Minutes*.

When race morning came, I arrived late to the start. It was a cold, drizzling day, and I was unprepared and inattentive. I remember tying my shoes and losing track of time. I got in my car to keep warm as all the other runners huddled together at the line. Then the gun fired, and I decided to jump out of my car and sprint to the start. This was, of course, inane. I must have had a sense that, somehow, the body had a separate tank for marathon energy that would replenish when I got to the start, the way children claim they have a second stomach for dessert. Off I went: shoes driving into the ground, water splashing upward.

Things went reasonably smoothly for remarkably long. A 22-year-old body can be pretty strong, even without proper care. I passed 20 miles in 2 hours and 20 minutes, just about on pace for a sub-three. I didn't know how I was supposed to feel, though. I hadn't trained my body for anything like this.

Then my stomach started to churn. I didn't know this then, but running hard is bad for the gut. We bounce up and down, jarring the stomach and the colon, and the body diverts blood away from the digestive system. It's a recipe for constant discomfort and occasional disaster. At about mile 22, I veered into the woods to relieve myself, and, when I returned to the road, I felt like my knees were the rusted hinges on a ladder long forgotten behind the barn. Neither my body nor my brain was prepared for this level of exhaustion. I finished in 3 hours and 18 minutes and then huddled miserably under a blanket, next to a long plastic table covered in discarded plastic cups. I don't remember how long I stayed. But eventually, a mess of grimy sweat partially rinsed by rainwater, I climbed into my battered Honda, which my father had bought for $12 and given to me. I drove to New York to begin my new life.

■

When I look back at that first marathon, I see so much that I did wrong, starting with the warm-up. I knew back then how to get ready for a track meet: jog, stretch, run some sprints. You need to get your heart rate up and your muscles warm. You need to expand your range of motion, and you need to activate the neural pathways you use when you run. You need to be relaxed but also ready to go hard off the starting line.

The marathon requires a different kind of warm-up, largely because it's an event with bewitching math. Your body goes fastest when it's burning carbohydrates, not proteins or fats. If you down your linguine properly before race day, you can store about 2,000 calories in carbs. Most of this energy is held as glycogen in your muscles, with a smaller amount in your liver. But 2,000 calories is not enough. You burn about 100 calories each mile you run, which means you can end up like me, in Rhode Island, wrecked and ravaged when there's still six miles to go. Runners call this "bonking," "hitting the wall," "blowing up," having "the piano on your back," and going into "zombie mode." It happens a lot.

There are strategies to counter this, starting with taking in carbohydrates as you run—drinking energy drinks or sucking down sweet, sticky, sickly blobs of carbohydrate gel. But the simplest thing is not to do what I did in Rhode Island and burn precious carbohydrate stores screwing around at the start. Now, to warm up for a marathon, I do almost nothing. I often sit near the start reading a magazine or newspaper that I can throw away. I try to lower my heart rate and relax my mind. I drink water and eat bananas and, usually, a bagel with peanut butter. Eventually, I get up, walk, and maybe jog for a minute. Then I amble over to the start.

Eventually, it's time to go. And this is where the most important lesson comes: slow down. At the start, one feels part of a flock of seagulls soaring up together after resting on a beach. Everything feels easy, and running fast feels free. You're surrounded by people, often by friends, and it's a relief finally to move after standing still. You might well have been cold, and now you'll be warm. But if it's a release, it needs to be a controlled one. It's tempting to run 5 seconds faster than your goal pace now, but you'll pay at least 10, and maybe 100, seconds a mile later. Success requires discipline of a peculiar type: the discipline not to push yourself too hard. The moment you speed up, a series of baleful chemical processes begins in the body. Hydrogen ions increase, causing the body's pH level to drop. The neural pathways with which our brains tell our bodies to move start to fray. Small tears begin to accumulate in the muscles, particularly in the quadriceps that we engage to keep us from tumbling forward as we run downhill.

Discipline isn't enough, though. You need to cultivate something else in these miles: awareness. The central challenge in marathoning is making sure your body is in balance. In a perfect race, you're running a steady pace, you're keeping steady form, and you understand how your body feels. In these early miles, if anything feels hard at all, anything at all, you have to slow down. The signals may be weak and easy to ignore—your heart might be beating just a touch too quickly or you may be breathing just a tiny bit hard—but they convey real danger. You need to hold this calm and relaxed pose as long as possible.

I didn't know any of this back then. I didn't know how to train. I didn't know how to warm up. And I didn't know what to do when things started to go wrong. I got 20 good miles in on that rainy day in Rhode Island because I was young and strong, because I had been fortunate in my genes, and because I had run all those mountains five years before. The last few miles, hobbling bow-legged in the cold, were what I deserved.

■

My early foray into the working world was equally inauspicious and for similar reasons. A few days after the marathon, in the fall of 1997, I showed up for my job at CBS as an associate producer in a new, ill-fitting Brooks Brothers suit. Upon arrival, I was summoned into the office of Phil Scheffler, the executive editor of the show. He had a short white beard and a bald, egg-shaped head. He'd been at the network since 1951, and he wanted to know who I was and why I had darkened the door of this place. I smiled and handed him a résumé that listed my college accomplishments and a couple of op-eds that I'd published in national newspapers during the past year.

I didn't realize that Scheffler was chopping my head off until it was halfway gone. He was skeptical and then a little condescending. He told me that the job of associate producer was a serious one for people with real experience in reporting, which I didn't have. He told me that I wasn't going to work there and pointed me toward the elevators. I was fired. I rode down and walked out into the cold sunny streets of Manhattan's

West Side. I looked at my watch. I had lasted precisely 59 minutes.

One of my closest friends was about to set out on a trip to West Africa. I decided, on a whim, to join him and to try my hand as a freelance foreign correspondent. My mother, following her normal philosophy of protecting me as well as she could while also granting me freedom, helped me figure out the relevant vaccinations and bought my plane ticket. I then spent the next few months bouncing around the continent by bus, staying in hostels, and observing a part of the world I had never visited before. It was a period of adventure and mishap. At one point, I was kidnapped by drug dealers in Morocco, who held me for 24 hours before deciding I would be useless as an international drug mule. My father had spent part of his first African sojourn in a Ghanaian jail; I spent part of mine locked in a bathroom outside of Tangier.

Four months later, after continuing through the continent and then traveling to Southeast Asia, I came back and started to work with my father on a book about the comparative economic trajectories of Ghana and Thailand. It wasn't easy. The man I knew as an adult lacked almost all discipline. We lived at the farm in Virginia and I worked in the office upstairs in a loft filled with photos of his years in the Reagan Administration. Settling myself on the black-and-white-striped couch coated entirely in reddish fur from our Irish setters, I'd pile up books, take notes, and type away. Then I'd look over the ledge to see what my father was up to on the floor below. Invariably, he was at his laptop, surfing porn or sexting with young men from across the world. Often there'd be a glass of cheap wine nearby. I'd tell him that we had to finish a chapter that day, and he'd promise that he'd get right on it. I'd look down again

20 minutes later and his screen would be filled with pictures, not words. It drove me crazy. We eventually got the manuscript done but, unsurprisingly, it wasn't very good.

■

My father wasn't an easy man to work with. But he sure was fun to live with because the traffic lights in his head were always green. He didn't like to sit still, because there was always something to do. He left parties, dinners, and movies when he was bored but never because he was tired. Hiking to the top of a mountain was always better than turning around. An argument was better than an agreement. I once brought a stray dog into the house and told my dad I was adopting it. He didn't even shrug. Nor did he shrug, a week later, when it ran away. My father believed in experience, and the more the better. My entire life, I never worried about waking him up when I called, because he was always awake.

We shared a love of music as well. When I was a child, he quizzed me on the characters in Mozart's operas and took me to the Boston Pops. All I need to hear are the few notes of Brahms's Piano Trio Number 1 in B Major and I'm back at the farm in Virginia. My father wanted to learn too. When we drove together, we'd alternate cassettes of Bach cantatas and free-jazz mixes my friend Taylor had sent me. Dad loved my weird instrumental acoustic guitar albums and gave them to all his friends.

When we lived together in Washington, while writing the book and then a year later, after I was hired as an editor at *The Washington Monthly*, we hosted countless parties together. I would invite my friends: young reporters, ambitious government officials, journalistic mentors. He would invite his: older intelligence operatives, congressmen, former students from abroad stationed in Washington, men he'd met that morning on the internet. Sometimes he would hire a cheap string quartet; sometimes, I would give impromptu concerts on my guitar. At one of the first parties, at his house just off Rock Creek Park, two of my female friends—whom I shall keep anonymous because they both went on to have successful careers in the United States government—showed up dressed only in Saran Wrap. We were always joined by Timothy Dickinson, a rumpled Oxford friend of my father's with a photographic memory who could multiply seven-digit numbers in his head and who served as something like a human encyclopedia for *Washington Post* columnists who wanted to appear more erudite—though his habit of drinking wine by the bottle made him unwelcome in some polite corners of the city. On election eve in 2000, we had probably 100 people in our house, evenly split between Bush and Gore supporters, until at least six in the morning. I remember falling asleep on the floor of the TV room, face-first without a pillow, wondering why my dad still had the book *The Married Homosexual Man* on his shelf. Timothy had passed out on a couch somewhere. Dad was sitting on his black Eames chair with a young, gay Caribbean diplomat on his lap watching the returns from Florida. We served cheap wine by the jug and cold pizza out of the box, but the house was always full. Washington elites were always happy to trade culinary indignities for a chance to debate hanging chads.

We weren't running much together, though. My father's body was like an old BMW, driven too hard, too long, and into too many trees. We could jog three or four miles, but rarely more. I bought him a book by Hal Higdon on how to train as a masters runner, but I don't think he ever opened it. I do remember him once telling me that he was resolved to get back at it. We were at his farm in Warrenton, Virginia, a nest of dog fur and sticky flytraps packed with victims hanging grotesquely from the ceiling. He put on his shorts and shoes, and I put on mine. Pamela, my little sister's elderly Irish setter, was lying on the couch. "What are you going to do: stay home and knit?" my father said in a teasing voice. She jumped up and bounded out the door with us.

We ran up the driveway, past the peach trees and the dozens of poplar trees we had planted up the whole side of the road. We turned and ran through the farm country, toward the cow pastures. After a mile or two, though, we turned around, and he said he needed to walk back. He weaved through the flytraps into the kitchen, where he poured himself his favorite recovery drink: a glass of orange juice and seltzer water.

■

When you train seriously as a runner, you realize two wonderful things: you can't get faster by magic, and you do get faster with effort. There are ways to optimize and to train smarter. And there are times when you work and work and don't get the result you want. But really, to get faster, particularly in a long race like a marathon, you have to get out every day and run—even when you're sore, tired, cold, grumpy, busy, or all of the above. You have to run when you have problems with aches, blisters, cramps, diarrhea, exhaustion, fasciitis, grogginess, headaches, ingrown toenails, jock itch, knee pain, lightheadedness, menstruation, numbness, overheating, panic, queasiness, rashes, swelling, toothaches, unhappiness, vomit, wounds, and xanthomas. You may have to run through swarms of yellowjackets, and you definitely have to run when you're zonked. One of the most important things to do in training for a marathon is, of course, to do long runs. Build up on weekends until you get to, say, 22 miles. But the deeper truth about training for a marathon is that you have to learn to run when you hurt, and you have to learn to hurt when you run. You have to learn to enjoy the pain.

You have to convince yourself over and over that the goal is worth the struggle. You have to run when you don't want to, and you have to do the extra loop around the lake when everything is telling you to go back home. You have to believe in the process. You have to believe that brick by brick, run by run, your body and mind are getting stronger. You have to believe this on days when you run slower than you did the week before. And if you want to run faster than you did before, you have to strain your body more than you did before. You have to build resilience so you can push yourself even more the next time you run. You have to search for that mystical sensation—the crux of this sport—where pleasure and pain blur into one. When you get there, pain means progress and progress means pleasure.

There are costs, of course. I've never met the spouse of a marathoner who has unambiguously positive feelings about their partner's sport. (Asked if she wanted to include a quote in this paragraph, Danielle smiled and tellingly demurred.) Marathon training can drain and distract you. It can open your mind and make you generous and gentle, but it can also make you self-absorbed and selfish. There are few things more boring at a cocktail party than a runner talking about his resting heart rate. Distance running also takes a lot of time if you want to do it right. For everyone who commits to long races, there's a set of trade-offs that have to be made and deals with friends and family that have to be struck.

My father often talked about momentum in life. Sometimes you have it; each success makes the next success a little easier and a little more likely. Sometimes you don't, and your losses compound. When you have it, he would tell me, keep it and use it. Focus. Get more done. Take the confidence that this success gives you and use it. When you don't have it, he'd say, well, try to get it back. This isn't bad advice, because every time we do something, we create grooves in our minds that make it easier to do the same thing again. It's how we learn to press our fingers to make a G chord on the guitar, how we learn to sit up straight at the dinner table, and how we learn to quit drinking—or how we get in the habit of drinking to deal with stress. When we have momentum, our habits seem to continually push us in the right direction. When we don't, it's often because our habits are pushing us the other way. It's a depressing thought because it means that each thing that goes wrong makes everything else, forever into the future, more likely to go wrong. Until we realize that the opposite is also true. Each time we do something right, we create a tiny imperceptible tailwind for the future.

I think of this often when I head out for a run. To have run during a day is to at least have done that. As my father descended into mania, the days when he ran were the days he kept everything else in control. If he had run more, could he have done more? When I was a child, there were days when I woke up and wished he hadn't already put on his sneakers and left the house. Now, looking back, I wish he had kept doing it for longer.

As my 20s progressed, I kept registering for marathons, always with the goal of breaking three hours but never with the knowledge of how to do it. I signed up for five, started four, completed three, and came within half an hour of my goal in two. In only one did I run the entire way. The worst was the 2003 New York City Marathon. I knew I needed to run 6:51 per mile, and I stayed on pace until the Bronx. By mile 23, as the race neared Central Park, I knew I wasn't going to make it. I was running 7:15 or 7:30 per mile. My knee hurt. I looked toward the trees in the park and the street in front of me. A friend of mine on a cargo bicycle yelled encouragement from the side of Fifth Avenue, but I just shook my head. My father and Danielle were at the finish line, three miles away.

I slowed to a walk, picked it up to a trot, and then stopped. Then I bent my head in shame, hoping no one who knew me was in the crowd, and walked off the course toward the 6 train. Dad and Danielle waited, confused, at the finish, watching streams of other runners cross the line. Eventually, I got word to them that I had gone home. They told me it was the right decision—what else could they say? But I knew it wasn't. My knee did hurt. But something always hurts that late in a marathon. I quit because I was afraid to fail, and my knee gave me an excuse. It turned out to be the only time my father came to one of my marathons, and I gave up.

My professional life was the same goat rodeo as my running. I had fallen in love with journalism. But journalism hadn't fallen in love with me. Everyone worked at *The Monthly* for two years. After my term was up, I moved back to New York to live with Danielle. I was rejected from dozens of full-time jobs and was struggling as a freelancer to find meaningful work. I compensated by making hundreds of dollars a day playing guitar on the platforms of the L train. But I knew I couldn't keep doing that, so I wrote countless job memos. I took part-time jobs as auditions. I took freelance assignments that required waking up at 2 A.M. I remember calling my mother on a pay phone and crying while explaining my latest setbacks. I finally got a wonderful job—as an editor at a magazine called *Legal Affairs*—but it was in New Haven, far from Danielle. We were married now, but she was dancing in New York and that was where we wanted to build our life. My worst moment came when I submitted a guest essay to *The Washington Monthly*. One of the editors sent me helpful feedback but mistakenly included the office's email chain about the story. In the part I wasn't meant to see, one of my closest peers and friends in the industry had written a scathing assessment both of the story and of my general abilities. Maybe, I began to ask myself, I just wasn't good enough? I applied to law school and was admitted to NYU. I needed to do something new.

I kept running and, in the spring of 2005, I went to Hopkinton to try again to crack three hours in the Boston Marathon, but I got a cold a few days before the race. I was a mess of cramps, coughs, and chills, and I walked across the finish line in 3:46. I crossed the line with my hands on my hips and my head down. Next to me, an older woman crossed with her arms up in celebration. That's one beautiful thing about a marathon: any finishing time can be a tragedy or a triumph.

But I knew I could run faster. Four weeks later, I entered the Delaware Marathon, took a train south, and tried again. This time I did it right. I started out at a 6:45-per-mile pace and stayed steady as the course looped through downtown Wilmington. Even with a mile to go, I was terrified that I would fail: that my hips would freeze, that my knees would buckle, that my feet would break. Repeated failure is both a motivator and a demon. In this case, it drove me forward. Soon I could see the finish line and the race clock, with the seconds ticking up from 2:57. For eight years I had held the goal of breaking three hours in my mind. Now I had done it. I had finished 30 minutes behind the winner—a local running legend named Michael Wardian—but in seventh place out of 507 finishers. Afterward, I wrote my dad. He responded with a confusing story about being robbed, maxing out his credit card, and having a conflict at the passport office. But then added, "serious congrats on the marathon. the best Thompson time ever! love dad"

He was genuinely proud that I'd beaten his fastest finish, and he framed a photograph of me crossing the line with the time displayed. One of his great virtues was that he never competed with me or resented any success I had. He had seen the agony that his father's resentment caused. My father made many mistakes in his life, but this would not be one of them.

■

A few months after my triumph in the Delaware Marathon, I was set to start at NYU. Then an executive at *Wired* reached out and suggested I apply for a job as an editor. One of his writers had told him that I was actually pretty good. This was what I wanted: a great journalism job in New York. I wanted to keep trying to tell stories, to explore, to learn. I started to interview and could tell that they liked me. But I also knew I wasn't going to have an offer before matriculation at NYU. I would have to choose between a sure thing and an unknown.

I delayed the decision as long as I could. Then, one day in August, right before orientation, I ran up Cadillac Mountain in Maine. I left in the predawn darkness and forged into the woods, across the beds of pine needles, then up the lichen-covered rocks. I jumped over rotted logs and twisted roots. I held on to iron rungs pounded into the stone at the steepest parts, maneuvering up in a style halfway between mountain running and rock climbing. The spruce trees thinned out until just a few remained, wind-shorn and shrunken among the rocks. Running up that mountain, I felt as if I were heading into a telescope, with the ocean and the islands revealing themselves as I ascended.

The sun came up as I ran, casting light onto my right shoulder as I climbed. I made it to the top and stood in the middle of the panorama among the Maine blueberries. A man with an American flag on his hat and some stoned teenagers were nearby. The kids looked at me quizzically, like I'd materialized from the clouds. I looked out over the ocean, picked up a flat stone, and imagined throwing it down and watching it skip eastward across the Atlantic Ocean.

We make big decisions in mysterious ways. I like to make charts of advantages and disadvantages. I like to call people to talk things through. I feel like I'm ready to make a choice only when the people I call don't have anything new to add. I also make choices with my gut. This time I didn't decide until I was bouncing back down the mountain, on what must have been a 20-mile run. I came home and told Danielle that I was withdrawing from NYU. I had just done the hard thing of running up a mountain, and it had convinced me that I could do this much harder thing of betting on myself. If I didn't get the job at *Wired,* I'd write a book. Looking back, it was the kind of choice my father should perhaps have made. One of the letters from the dons at Oxford had perceptively noted that he was built more like a journalist—curious, gregarious, always moving—and that he didn't have the intense, singular focus of an academic.

When I came back from Maine, I was as strong as I'd been since college. I had spent eight years trying to run a three-hour marathon, and, once I did, I realized I could go much faster. I trained with new dedication and tracked my resting heart rate as it dropped by the day. That August I ran a half-marathon in 1:20. I got the *Wired* job. I wrote and sold a proposal for a book about the Cold War and the rivalry between George Kennan and my maternal grandfather, Paul Nitze. Brimming with confidence, I emailed a friend of mine from childhood, Margaret Angell, who had become a great runner. I asked for suggestions on getting even better, and she directed me to her running team, which met on Thursday nights at the statue of Daniel Webster near West 72nd Street in Central Park. I hadn't run with a team in a decade, but I started showing up every week. The coach, a chiseled, effervescent man named Tony Ruiz, gave us our workouts. Then he'd sprint across the park and find a spot to cheer us on. He told me that I ran with my arms too high, and he took delight in my improvements.

At work, on Thursday afternoons, I started to feel a bit as I had on race days at Andover. There was a pot inside me, overflowing with nervous energy. I feared failure; I craved success; I could imagine myself running as fast as everyone else; I could imagine myself falling off the pack. I woke up every morning wanting to run. My confidence rose. I started with the B group, and then eventually moved up to the A group. Setting off in the back of a cluster of maybe 10 runners, I'd usually find myself ending with two or three, dashing through the center of Central Park. The season was changing from summer to fall, and the leaves were turning the color of my new orange racing singlet. I'd pass the carriage horses, wondering whether any of them wanted to break free of their little buggies and run by my side.

I began doing long runs on weekends and found a favorite 20-mile loop: heading out on the Belt Parkway bike path from central Brooklyn to Coney Island. I'd run on the boardwalk past the aquarium and then down a little ramp to Ocean Parkway. From there, it was a straight six miles back to Prospect Park. Every time I ran at dawn through outer Brooklyn, at least one person would yell at me, "Run, Forrest, run."

In October, I took the ferry to Staten Island, where I ran a half-marathon in 1:15. I sent my splits to my father, noting that I had averaged 5:45 per mile. He didn't quite understand how good I'd become. My time in the Delaware Marathon meant I was fast; the gradations faster than that didn't compute to him. I knew, though. I must have refreshed the web page with my race results 20 times.

Everything was falling into place. Danielle was finishing her dissertation at NYU in the Performance Studies department. I adored my new colleagues at *Wired,* and I was starting to put the pieces of my book on the Cold War together. Danielle and I started to talk about having children. She would defend her dissertation in the spring; the right time to have a child would be the next fall. We could start trying, we thought, in December.

In November 2005, I ran the New York City Marathon in 2:43, putting me in 146th place out of 37,000 entrants. I realized that I had talent. I was starting to understand hard training. I figured I would keep going and get faster still. The Thursday after the marathon, I headed up to West 72nd Street to run again. Ruiz called my name out to all the runners in the circle and noted how much better I had gotten. He gripped my shoulder in a kind of masculine intimacy. The man was proud of me; he wanted to see more. All I wanted to do was race again. I had momentum and I wanted to get back out there. Just like my father had told me to do.

CHAPTER 6

Tony Ruiz

That's it. You can never do this again. You're going to die if you ever do.
—TONY RUIZ

TONY RUIZ KNEW HE WAS FAST WHEN HE WAS SEVEN YEARS OLD. He went to school on Manhattan's Lower East Side, on East 10th Street and Avenue D, and every day he'd race a kid named Harold Vasquez to the building. People would cheer them on from the street, but Ruiz lost and lost and lost until one day he didn't. This gave him confidence, and he never lost again.

Ruiz was born in 1961 in Spanish Harlem, but his family moved around a lot. At Mark Twain Intermediate School in Coney Island, he started to run track. He was a sprinter at first, but his coach decided that Ruiz might have talent for longer distances. There wasn't a measured track nearby, so the coach just pointed at a tree and told Ruiz to run to it and back. Ruiz, it turned out, had the genes for endurance. Soon he was running the half-mile, and he won every time. In the city championship, as an eighth grader, he won while wearing ragged PRO-Keds against a group of kids who wore racing shoes with spikes, which Ruiz had never seen before.

In 1976, when Ruiz was a high school sophomore at Westinghouse in Downtown Brooklyn, he went to see the Penn Relays, one of the biggest track meets in the country. His coach, who called him Ton-yah, told him to go and watch the distance medley relay. It was all skinny white kids, except for one skinny Black kid named Maurice Weaver. Weaver and his team swept to victory. "That was significant to me," Ruiz remembers. It was the moment when he realized that Black and Hispanic guys could be distance runners, not just sprinters. Later that sophomore year, Ruiz told his coach that there was another kid at the school who could beat him: a lean, quiet Black kid named Billy Pearson who loved to play basketball. "Ton-yah," his coach said, "if that's true, we are going to be one of the greatest teams ever assembled. But I don't believe you." Ruiz took his coach to the lunchroom, where Billy was sitting by himself. "You think you can beat Ton-yah?" the coach asked. "Yeah," Billy responded.

Billy joined the team that afternoon and had no problem keeping up on an 8-mile jog. Soon he was winning races. He and Ruiz led one of the best high school teams New York had ever seen. They won multiple city and state titles. Their two-mile relay team was ranked top in the nation by *Track & Field News*.

Ruiz was the team captain. He was tough and a little bit wild. He smoked more weed than is recommended for a high school track athlete. But he missed only one workout in his four years on the team. (He had failed a class, so his mother made him stay home, where he spent the day sprinting up and down the stairs.) Running was his life and, he later reflected, part of what saved him from the gangs that ran his part of Brooklyn.

In the fall of 1976, Ruiz ran a cross-country meet on a Saturday. A friend and teammate, Louis Jimenez, had crashed at his place, and they planned to run about 15 miles the next day. They got up early and saw on television that the New York City Marathon was happening and that it would start in a few hours in Staten Island. They hopped on a bus and made their way across the Verrazzano.

This was the seventh year of the marathon, but the first time it traversed all five boroughs. There's a photograph of the start of that race and, off to the left, you can see young Ruiz in a yellow Westinghouse singlet, without a number, heading off the line. He has thick arms and legs, and a short Afro. He and Jimenez ran steadily at sub-6-minute pace, keeping in a pack with a five-foot-tall, 90-pound Japanese-American named Miki Gorman, who would win the women's race. In one photo taken on the course, Ruiz and Jimenez are barreling along Fourth Avenue in Brooklyn, right in front of Gorman and a man with a receding hairline dressed improbably in white khaki pants and a collared shirt. Jimenez and Ruiz eventually slowed a little. But as they approached the finish line, they started to sprint. A security guard noticed that they didn't have race numbers, and he jumped out from the sidelines and knocked them both to the ground.

■

Ruiz's mother had gotten the family out of the projects. She worked hard as a cleaning lady and kept good credit. His stepdad worked as an elevator operator and saved his money too.

"We are in Brighton Beach in a fucking house, you see?" Ruiz told me. "And it's not a coincidence that my four brothers and sisters, we're all still alive. All our friends, they're dead."

Billy Pearson couldn't get out. High school and the track had given him structure. It had sheltered the quiet, introspective boy. But when high school ended, life got hard. Billy had grown up in the Howard Houses projects in Brownsville, one of the toughest neighborhoods in New York. "He's from the projects, man. His dad was never there. I think he was a bus driver. He never came to the meets," Ruiz said. "So, it's a story of how the streets will swallow your ass up."

At age 19, Billy was arrested for gun possession and spent a year in prison. When he came out, he had lost his love for running and, seemingly, everything else. Billy had joined the Nation of Islam for protection on the inside, and, now, Ruiz said, "he owed people." Ruiz tried to convince him to stay with the sport, but Billy told him he was done. The quiet, introspective young man became a gangster. A few years later, he dropped his ID while stealing furniture. The cops recovered it, and Billy realized he was going to go back to prison. Ruiz isn't sure what happened next. He heard a story that Billy drank hydrochloric acid and declared that he would never again go to jail. Then he ran toward the hospital screaming in pain saying he needed help. The acid had already eaten through his system, and he couldn't get there fast enough. He died at the age of 24.

■

After graduating from high school in 1979, Ruiz moved to San Juan to go to the University of Puerto Rico in Bayamón. He hadn't been particularly serious about his academics, but his track coach had managed to adjust his transcript enough for him to get in. The coach's view, Tony recalled, was that the world was so stacked against his kids that it was only fair to cheat a little bit on their behalf. Tony did interviews with Spanish-language radio stations and told them that he was going to make it to the Olympics.

When Ruiz was a year old, his parents had split and his biological father had moved to the island. He hadn't supported his son, and he hadn't responded when his son once wrote for help to buy racing spikes. Still, Ruiz's father showed up for the first big cross-country college race and infuriated Ruiz by telling him before the start how good the local runners were. Ruiz, a freshman running against hundreds of older boys in unfamiliar heat and humidity, ended up coming in second. When he finished, his father was in tears. "Now you know who I am," Ruiz said. "And who I became when you didn't send me spikes."

The rest of the year, Ruiz was a dynamo. He quickly beat the junior national champion. He was undefeated on the track. He was certain he would make the 1980 Puerto Rican Olympic team. But Puerto Rico wouldn't go that year. The Games were to be held in Moscow, and Jimmy Carter had withdrawn the U.S. team because of the Soviet invasion of Afghanistan. Puerto Rico, which fields its own team, decided not to send its runners. A few days later, Ruiz attended a dinner hosted for the athletes who would likely have made the team and was given a beautiful inscribed Bulova watch.

Shortly thereafter, Ruiz bolted. If he wasn't going to be in the Olympics, he wasn't going to stay on the island. He left school without telling his coach and moved back to New York, where he got a job working in the mail room at Rockefeller Center. But without the structure of his running life and the

Olympics to aim for, he started doing crack. In December 1980, he went to a Christmas party at Rockefeller Center and wore his watch to impress his colleagues. He had much too much to drink and stumbled back toward home via the subway. When he got off at Coney Island at about 1 A.M., he decided he wanted to find a female companion. He walked down Ocean Parkway and toward the ramp that takes you up to the boardwalk. As he approached, two guys grabbed him. One of them put a knife to his neck. They took his wallet, his money, his chain, his coat, and his watch. Then they grabbed the ring off his finger. "The thing that got me cut was my damn high school ring, man," Ruiz recalls. "I didn't want to give that up. They were trying to get my fucking ring, my Westinghouse ring, the high school ring. Dude, I fucking caught that guy so good in his jaw. I nailed him."

The muggers broke off, holding the ring, and sprinted up the ramp and out onto the boardwalk to the aquarium. The knife had sliced into Ruiz's neck just above the jugular, but the blade was sharp, and he didn't feel it. He was about to race off after them when two men appeared. "Hey, we saw everything that happened. Let's go to the hospital," one of them said. "I'm looking at them like, 'Nah, nah. I'm going to catch those motherfuckers.' Then the guy said, 'No, no, you got to go to the hospital,'" Ruiz recounted. One of the men took off his own jacket and used it to slow the bleeding from Ruiz's neck. On the way, they passed a bar that Ruiz knew, and he belligerently insisted they go in. The owner, an Italian man named Alfie, took one look at Ruiz and sent him away. "Tony, I'm not serving you a fucking beer. Get to a goddamn hospital." When he finally got there, the doctor told him that if he had tried to chase the two men down, he would almost certainly have bled to death on the boardwalk. He still has the scar.

Ruiz returned to running even as his drug habit worsened. In 1981, he entered the New York marathon, not having run more than 10 miles on any day in a year. He finished in 2:34 and, afterward, joined the Central Park Track Club, one of the largest and strongest teams on the East Coast. He qualified for the Puerto Rican national championships at 1500 meters but suffered every runner's nightmare. When the 1500-meter runners were called to the start over the stadium loudspeakers, Ruiz had his headphones on, listening to Michael Jackson's *Off the Wall*. He was stretching with his back to the track and turned around to see his rival, Jorge "Yoyo" Ortiz, rounding the first curve. The race had begun without him.

One year, he entered a five-mile turkey trot in Prospect Park. He spent the night before with a girlfriend on Parkside Avenue doing cocaine and didn't sleep a single minute. He showed up hungover and high, but still fit. About three and a half miles in, right before the course turned up a big hill, Ruiz pulled to the side and threw up. He told one teammate he was dropping out. Then another of his teammates ran by, a guy named Barry who Ruiz had never been fond of and who he called "sort of an entitled white dude." The idea of losing to Barry sobered Ruiz right up, and he got back on the course. He raced up the hill, passed Barry on the descent, and finished in a bit over 25 minutes.

Ruiz married a woman named Charlene, but life just kept getting worse. He sold his TV and stereo for crack and tried to convince Charlene that the house had been robbed. He tried to kill himself by jumping off the terrace of a 13th-floor apartment, but only one leg cleared the barrier. Finally, one morning after he had spent the night in a Harlem crack house, he broke down on 126th Street, bankrupt and despondent. He and Charlene now had a very young son, and Tony knew he needed to get straight. He started to walk toward the hospital when he saw a dollar in the street and picked it up. He knew he should use it to get some fruit; he hadn't eaten in a while. Instead, he bought a Budweiser. At that moment, he remembers thinking, *Wow, Tony. You are a really sick guy. God put that dollar in your path.* He downed the beer and declared it was the last one he would ever have. He walked straight to the rehab center at Gracie Square Hospital.

I asked Ruiz whether he was thinking about his family that morning when he entered rehab. "You can't just do it for other people. It has to come from within," he responded. "And that's why I say when I walked with that dollar and bought that last beer, I could feel like there was something more powerful than me that was telling me, 'This is it, Tony.' And it wasn't my mother. I wasn't thinking about my son at the time. It was just like a moment that I had with my higher power that just told me, 'That's it. You can never do this again. You're going to die if you ever do this thing, drink or drug, again.' And I haven't done it since April 15, 1988."

■

Ruiz joined Alcoholics Anonymous and redirected his energy into staying clean. He came back to running after taking a year and a half off, but getting sober took the edge off. He didn't have the same desire to beat everyone anymore. He had run fast when he was young, partly because he was mad at the world. Now he had changed. "When you get in recovery, you mellow out. All the goodness in you comes out," he says. He was trying to find himself, trying to be a good father. "I just wanted to focus on staying alive."

One day, a man in his building in East New York told Ruiz that he looked like a serious runner and asked if he would coach his local girls' team. Ruiz turned three of them into city champions. Soon, the coach of the Central Park Track Club asked Ruiz to be an assistant. Six years later, he became the head coach.

Ruiz was now coaching college stars who had just moved to the city; recreational runners who realized they had talent; masters athletes who hadn't missed a day of running in 30 years; and bankers who had done well in a Corporate Challenge race. The team was mostly white Manhattan professionals. When they went to prison, it was for white-collar crime. It was the beginning of an era in which running evolved counter to most other social trends. As human attention spans became shorter and our phones began to buzz all the time, millions of people decided that they wanted to run 26.2 miles. The word "marathon" has mostly negative connotations, particularly when used as an adjective: "marathon commute," "marathon meeting," "marathon call." (Perhaps the only positive one is "marathon sex.") Culturally, though, running a marathon earned one cachet. In Ruiz's first year as a coach, the fastest marathoner for the club finished in 2:28. The slowest ran 5:47. Ruiz loved coaching them all.

Soon afterward, my friend Margaret Angell, who had recently graduated from Harvard and was working in corporate finance, joined the team. She had just run a 3:16 marathon when she started coming to workouts with the club. Ruiz told her she could be great. He gave her structured workouts. He instructed her to run with the men. By 2004, she had run a 2:47 marathon and had qualified for the Olympic Trials. She finished in 30th place at the Trials and set the club record in the process. It was, Ruiz said, the most rewarding experience in his years of coaching. A few months after that, Margaret emailed me and suggested I join the club.

Ruiz stayed on through my years and long after. But his coaching came to an end during the coronavirus pandemic. Ruiz understood the science, but there wasn't any way he was going to get a vaccine injection. "I'm in recovery, dude. I don't take flu shots. I don't take anything I don't have to take," he said. "God has given me this fucking opportunity and I commit."

This was the period when vaccination had become a tribal issue in America, and the club wasn't sympathetic to Ruiz's position. He tried to compromise, committing to wearing a mask at practice. But he suffers from asthma, and one day, at practice out in Central Park, he took his mask down. A woman on the team came over to chastise him. Ruiz stood up here, irate at the memory. "She comes over to me like I'm a three-year-old kid; she's like, 'What are you doing?'"

Ruiz's voice then gets high and whiny as he re-creates the moment, "'Your mask, your mask. You got to put your mask on. You got to put your mask on.' People are right there. Embarrassing me. So then, I looked at her. I said, 'You mean this?' I fucking flung it to the ground. I fucking left." That was it. Soon, Ruiz was done coaching for the team.

He's still running, though, and in fact he's back with an intensity he hasn't had since before he got clean. He's now in his early 60s, trying to set masters records and age-graded personal bests. He's back out there, going for it all, just as he did more than 50 years ago on Avenue D.

CHAPTER 7

Falling Apart at Forty

Death is very likely the single best invention of life. It is Life's change agent.... Your time is limited, so don't waste it living someone else's life.

—STEVE JOBS, STANFORD COMMENCEMENT ADDRESS, 2005

TWO WEEKS AFTER COMPLETING MY TRIUMPHANT NEW YORK CITY Marathon in 2005, I saw my doctor for my annual physical. He took the usual measurements and ran through the usual routine. Then he put his fingers on my throat to check for lumps. He lingered a little longer than normal on one spot. "There's something there," he said. He told me that it could be a cyst, which would be fine, or a nodule, which might not.

I didn't worry much. I had just run a fast marathon. I had always eaten a lot of spinach and hydrated well. I had many insecurities, but my health was not one of them. Gradually, though, the prognosis darkened. A sonogram determined it was a nodule, not a cyst. I traveled through hospitals for tests in blue gowns, each time certain that the next result would vindicate my assumption that the lump was just a benign biological blip of some kind. I was only 30, after all.

Each test result only worsened the forecast and darkened my odds. Eventually the doctors determined that the only option available was surgery. An aptly named Dr. Cutter would have to open my neck to figure out what this little lump really was. I was deep in research for my book about the Cold War and felt particularly remiss that my own medical woes forced me to cancel two interviews that I'd scheduled with nonagenarians.

My mother came to New York, and she and Danielle took me to NYU Hospital for my surgery. The procedure was horrifying: the doctors would be nearly cutting off my head. But it was also a simple process and I'd be unconscious. My mother and Danielle would have the harder task of waiting, wondering, worrying. Eventually my name was called. I was given the anesthesia, and for a brief moment I tried to concentrate on the surgeons, hoping I could somehow supervise the task. Then the lights went out.

My father was the parent people thought would be president. But he would have melted down at the first reports that the embassy in Tehran had been stormed. Stress made him short-circuit. He couldn't talk about the cancer, and he certainly couldn't offer any help. He started drinking more, worrying more, and writing me less. He later told me that he had become convinced I would die.

My mother, meanwhile, was like a reverse transformer. Small voltage shifts or tiny bits of stress—like making sure someone had put the potatoes in the oven on time—could overwhelm her circuits. Actual catastrophes, like my illness, seemed to make her calmer and more in control. She made me feel that she would have given up anything if it meant that I would live for one more day.

Dr. Cutter removed half of my thyroid gland. I felt nauseated afterward, and I wasn't allowed to exercise for three weeks. I had the scar of a necklace, which I'll have as a marker for the rest of my life. My neck felt out of balance, like I was a strawberry with the stem partly cut off. I waited a week for the lab results. Then one day, while I was in New Hampshire with friends, I got the call. The tumor was benign. I told Danielle and gave her a hug. You learn a lot about how someone feels about you when you see their face at the exact instant of your triumph or despair. I have never seen anyone as happy as Danielle was then.

Two weeks later, I got a second, crushing phone call: the first group of doctors had read the slide wrong, and a review team had determined that I did have thyroid cancer. It was an eminently treatable variant, with a survival rate over 90 percent. But it was still cancer. I told Danielle, and we went for a walk in the cold Brooklyn air.

In short order, I would need a second surgery to get the rest of the thyroid out. My neck already felt vulnerable. Now they would have to cut again. My surgeons were gentle and kind people, but as I went under anesthesia, I worried that they would just finish all the business while I was there and do what the French swordsman had done to Anne Boleyn. My mother came down for this surgery too.

After the second operation, I was miserable. Without my thyroid, I felt dizzy constantly and couldn't regulate my temperature. I felt cold when others felt warm. My tendons hurt. I got headaches all the time. Then I had to prepare for a radiation treatment, which meant going on a low-iodine diet and taking two doses of rectal suppositories to empty out my system. After the treatment I would need to quarantine alone for a week at home. I told my boss, but I tried to hide my diagnosis from my colleagues at *Wired*, most of whom worked in San Francisco. I told none of my new friends on the Central Park Track Club; I just didn't show up at workouts anymore. I desperately wanted to keep things as normal as I could.

Danielle and I got our apartment ready. We set out plastic silverware and put everything I thought I would need in one room so that I wouldn't even need to go into the other ones. I moved the philodendron and the other houseplants into the room I wouldn't be using. Then I bicycled to the hospital in midtown Manhattan, where I was given a radioactive pill to swallow. It felt oddly normal for such a grave circumstance—like taking a multivitamin that came packed in an imposing lead container. But once I had swallowed it, I was a moving radiation site. I had to leave quickly, get on my bicycle, and try to stay as far away as possible from everyone else as I pedaled back home to Brooklyn. Danielle, who was just two weeks away from defending her dissertation, moved in with friends. Every day, she would come by our apartment and drop off soup for me at the door.

I spent a week alone as the radiation moved through my body, hunting down the cancerous cells. I was caged and despairing. I tried to stay calm, and I kept doing my job at *Wired*, editing stories by email. But I wasn't just dealing with pain; I was confronting death in a way that I hadn't had to before. Every now and then, I would go for short walks by myself, keeping far away from other people. I carried a note in my pocket from a doctor in case I got pulled over by a policeman with a Geiger counter.

We all, of course, are dying every day. However you do the math, we aren't around for very long: most of us live only for approximately 80 years, 4,000 weeks, or 2.5 billion seconds. Most of the time it's simpler to assume immortality than to do the calculations. Alone in a portion of our one-bedroom apartment, with radiation ripping my body apart, the calculations forced themselves on me. Death was no longer just an intellectual exercise. Five months ago, I had been a sub-elite marathoner; now, as I lay in agony on the red rug, I felt like that man had melted. I had been torn apart, and it was all because of a cluster of cells I could neither see nor feel.

The week ended, though, as I knew it would. It felt, I wrote to a friend, like the winter solstice: the evenings were still dark, but now every day would get lighter. I deep-cleaned the apartment with the windows wide open and Danielle came back. More scans made clear that the cancer was gone. Now I could begin the process of recovering. My diagnosis had come right after my triumphant marathon, and I believed that the only way to put it in the past was to run again. Odysseus had to string his old bow and fire an arrow through 12 axe heads to prove that he was the man he had once been. I needed to run another marathon.

I gradually started to train. My new medications made me perpetually dizzy, and I had to progress slowly from walking to bicycling to running. I had lost my strength and some of my coordination. My body had once seemed like a finely tuned instrument; now sometimes it would slide wildly out of key. I'd run two miles into the park and start to see double. I'd stop, and trudge slowly back. But I kept progressing, stubbornly and steadily. I became stronger, and I began to remember what it felt like to go fast. One glorious day that summer, I ran 10 miles in Brooklyn and talked with Danielle about having children. Not long after that, I ran 15 miles in the mountains of Aspen; tears and sweat dripped down my face as I came down Smuggler Mountain Road back into town.

As I healed, cancer went from the only thing I thought about, to something I thought about all the time, to something I thought about once a day, to something I could put to the side. When I did come back to it, I was often running. And then, two years after the diagnosis, I finished that New York City Marathon 13 seconds faster than I had before I got sick. I teared up again at the finish and then again a month later, when Tony Ruiz gave me the "comeback of the year" award at our track team's annual dinner. He gave me a hug and told me that he knew I'd been through a lot. I didn't know back then how much that meant.

■

By the time I ran the next marathon, I was a father. Ellis arrived in the summer of 2008. Danielle went on tour in Europe with her modern dance company a month later, and I went with her, bringing Ellis to her rehearsals in a BabyBjörn strapped to my chest. He and I watched the election of Barack Obama in a bar in Leuven, Belgium. I sat on a stool drinking a Stella and told him, now four months old, that he should pay attention to history being made. Zachary arrived two years after that and James four years later. Each time, my mother came to New York immediately to help with the babies. Watching her handle them with ease, and with infinite wisdom, made me appreciate even more what she had done for me. She would later tell me that she was never more proud of me than when she realized how much I loved my children.

Parenthood focused my mind and changed every ring of our life. Our social circle narrowed; our careers gained direction. I had less time in my life, but I cared about everything more. I watched how the boys learned—observing, listening, mimicking—and tried to be as attentive as they were. I finished my book about the Cold War, and it was praised more than anything else I'd ever written. One of the stories I'd assigned and edited at *Wired* became the movie *Argo*, which won the Academy Award for Best Picture. I worked with two friends to create a multimedia magazine and software startup called *The Atavist* that got funded by some of the most prominent venture capitalists in the world. I started receiving job offers for positions from writer to TV host. For the next six years, I would join CNN International on Wednesday mornings to talk about tech. My father, 12 hours ahead in Asia, would gather his friends after dinner and watch.

I was never quite sure why so much changed for the better in these years, until one day, at an event in Montana, I was sitting in a bus with Arthur Brooks, an expert on happiness and an *Atlantic* contributor. I asked him to tell me the number-one predictor of happiness and satisfaction. "There's one thing you can do," he said. "What's that?" "Get cancer and survive it," he responded, unaware that I had ever been sick.

He pointed me to the research. Multiple studies have shown that survivors of cancer often experience what is known as post-traumatic growth. Standing on the edge of mortality gives them clarity about what matters. They now appreciate life more; they feel increasingly self-assured; they've confronted the fact that they don't have much time left, so they value it more.

Much of the data is self-reported, and it depends on whether someone fully recovers. But it was true for me. After I recovered, I cut some of the trivia out of my life. I'd wake up early and start work before everyone else got up. Then I'd run to the office for my day in the Condé Nast Building at 4 Times Square. I'd stash suits in a closet there and run in with a fanny pack holding my phone, wallet, and keys. I'd shower in a gym nearby and go to the office in my shorts—always hoping that I wouldn't end up in an elevator with Anna Wintour. Once at my desk, I'd work as intently as I could, knowing that I'd almost certainly leave at 6 P.M. to go home and play with the boys.

When I look back, I also see how I was learning to pace myself, both as a runner and as a journalist. I put aside all the stress I had carried in my 20s as I'd struggled to meet my father's professional expectations and my own. I was learning to just work hard and steadily and to trust that something good would happen next. And I was learning that everything came together better if I could find time to run and to think.

Sometimes, I would run on weekend nights at 11 P.M., after the kids and Danielle had gone to bed. I'd circle across the Williamsburg Bridge and pass the same East Village haunts where I'd performed on my guitar a decade before. I'd run out to Coney Island as the sun rose and watch the way my shadow would flow around me in a semicircle as I passed under each streetlight. When Zachary was a baby, I ran the New York City Marathon on almost no sleep. He had stayed up through the night, and I had kept him bouncing on my knee until it was time to head to the ferry. When I left, I handed him to Danielle.

I'd next see him, all bundled up in a stroller, on Atlantic Avenue.

It was in these years that I learned the most vital running lesson of my life. The weather is always good enough to run in, and there's always a spot to go. I'll run in 100-degree heat with ice tucked into my hat and when it's 15 below with Vaseline rubbed on my nose. I'll run in hail and in a dust storm. I'll run circles around a driveway or a parking lot if that's the only place to go. I've disobeyed a thousand no-trespassing signs and been chased by a dozen dogs, at least one cow, and a lemur. A cop in New Hampshire once called my running to a halt thinking I was a prison escapee. I've run through Times Square at midnight. I once ran around Las Vegas in shorts and a ski jacket because I forgot to bring a T-shirt on a trip. I've run to black-tie events with my tux in my backpack and changed in the men's room. I've jogged to airports and headed right to the security line.

Eventually, I got the one email I wanted, from an executive at *The New Yorker*, asking me to apply to become a senior editor. I focused and prepared. I sent over notes on roughly 20,000 words of draft articles. I sent ideas. I sat for hours of interviews. I made lists and practiced questions in my head. I knew I was doing well, but jobs like this aren't easy to get. Eventually, Pam McCarthy, the deputy editor, sent me the note I dreaded: my efforts were appreciated, but the job had gone to someone else. I soon learned that a highly respected book editor with a rather similar name, Nick Trautwein, had beaten me out.

A few months went by. Then in early December, I showed up at a holiday party and started talking to a young woman who was rather deep in her cups. She was an assistant at *The New Yorker*, close to the center of power. I told her my name, and she paused for a second. "Nick Thompson? Oh my god. They went back and forth, and back and forth. Thompson? Trautwein? Trautwein or Thompson? Thompson or Trautwein?" She swayed a little bit to the poetry of the diptych.

Coming close is painful. But it also gave me a reason to try again. Three months after the holiday party, I was about to leave *Wired* to take a job as a writer at another magazine. I was ready for a new challenge, and the role came with a substantial raise. I was about a week away from having to make the final decision when, in the strange, quiet morning hours of early parenthood, I pulled a thin volume off the shelves, *The Survival of the Bark Canoe*, by John McPhee. I read it straight through. It's the story of an obsessive, thoughtful man in southern New Hampshire who makes beautiful birch-bark canoes fashioned with traditional Native American tools. Eventually, he and the author travel up to the Allagash River in the north woods of Maine. It's a story with nary a plot twist, or even a dramatic scene. But every paragraph had something beautiful, something moving, something that seemed like an axe taken to the frozen waters inside me. McPhee had spent his working life at *The New Yorker*. That was the place I needed to be. I drafted McCarthy an email at about three in the morning saying that I was soon going to take a job at a rival publication, and that I would love another shot.

She wrote back and told me to come have lunch. We did, and then I took another edit test. I went to see David Remnick, the editor in chief. He didn't have much time, he said, so he was just going to be blunt. They hadn't hired me the first time because they feared my attention was scattered. The job wasn't for someone who would write, edit, go on TV, start companies on the side, and mess around with Hollywood. It was for someone who would sit at a desk and focus. Drafts would arrive at my desk. I would pick them up, read them, and do my best to make them better. That was the job. And I would do it for a long time. Could I promise him that I'd stay on task? Why, yes, I said, I could. Shortly afterward, I sent him an email. "I'm writing just to note one point. I'll be fine if you think I flopped the edit test, if there isn't really a spot, or if we can't work out the details. But I don't want to lose out because of a sense that I wouldn't work fiendishly hard as an editor, editor, editor." A few days later, I had the job.

■

My father was thrilled by my professional success, perhaps particularly because his life was unraveling. He had moved to Asia, going back and forth between the Philippines and Indonesia, when I was about 30. Once or twice a year, he would fly across the world, come to my apartment, and just empty his suitcase in the middle of the floor, spilling crumpled clothes, gin bottles, tubes of moisturizer, and unopened mail all over the place. He couldn't pay his bills. I don't know if he brushed his teeth. When he moved to Asia, he owed the IRS $338,000 and had an annual income—from his university pension and from a trust that my mother had set up for him after the divorce—of about a fifth of that.

He came to Brooklyn to visit soon after Ellis was born, and I was startled both by his obvious love and admiration for his grandchild and by his total incompetence. He didn't know how to hold a baby: trying to hoist Ellis, he looked like a man trying to lift a greasy turkey from the fridge. He had no idea of how to change a diaper, making me suspect that he had never changed mine. He came back when Zachary was born and then when James arrived. My father was full of admiration for the boys, but he came carting chaos. He'd say he had to step outside to buy aspirin, and then I'd find him smoking and slugging gin and orange juice on the front stoop. One morning, sitting in our apartment overlooking Grand Army Plaza, with piles of his scattered papers tossed upon our dinner table, he told me that his iPad had crashed and he needed me to fix it. I rebooted it, only to discover that he had been trying to schedule time with a male prostitute in our guest room after Danielle and I headed out for work. It hadn't occurred to my dad that the children, and their nanny, would still be there. I told him that I'd fixed the device but that he really shouldn't do the thing he'd just been doing. He declared that he hadn't been doing anything at all except working on an op-ed for *The Jakarta Post*. I said, "Don't lie to me," and then walked down the stairs and told the doorman to not let anyone in while I was gone. That night, I balanced a chair against my father's door in such a way that it would clatter if he headed out.

In 2013, my father planned a visit just as I was going to run the Brooklyn Marathon, a race of eight loops around Prospect Park. I had practically begged him to come to watch the race— I desperately wanted him to see me run fast at least once. But he couldn't make the logistics work. He showed up that afternoon, as I hobbled around the apartment with my aching post-marathon quads. He too was struggling to walk, having just had an operation on his hips. He told me that his struggles reminded him how important it is to remember a child's first steps. This time I put him in an Airbnb in a fancy building on Prospect Park West. It seemed like a success, and the host was delighted to have such a smart and worldly man in the apartment. On the final morning, though, I came to pick my father up, and he hurried out the door. He had become incontinent during the night, wasn't quite sure what had happened, and wanted to get out fast. I sent an extra-large tip.

In 2015, when I turned 40, my father put a note on my Facebook page that was visible to my friends and my then roughly 70,000 followers. I had a great life, he said: a loving wife, three beautiful children, a successful career. But all men's lives, he noted, fall apart at this age. He was 73 then, and he could look back at his own life, his peers', and, most important, his own father's. There's too much pressure and too many temptations, he said. He had entered a spiral at this age and had never quite recovered. He added that he hoped the same would not happen to me.

I read the note, puzzled. It was a private comment made in a very public place. I responded in a comment with goofy humor and deflection, but it made me realize something. I had spent much of my life trying to be like my father: going to the same schools, going to Africa, running, pursuing the same ambitions, forever seeking his approval. But I also desperately wanted not to be like him. I didn't want my discipline to drop. I didn't want to get knocked off-balance by life. I didn't want my id to overcome my superego. I didn't want my life to fall apart at 40. Running seemed like it might be the key. He had stopped. I was going to keep on doing it, and I was going to keep doing it well.

■

It sometimes seems like a miracle that humans can run at all. You crash your feet into the ground, one after the other, pushing down on the pavement. The force then rebounds through the tendons of the lower legs, propelling you forward through the air. You recruit muscle fibers to do this again and again. Meanwhile, stress is sent up your ankle, through your knees, across your hips, into your back. Your feet flex and your abdominal muscles try to keep you steady. Your arms swing, providing a dynamic and balancing force, but also putting stress on the shoulders. Your diaphragm works in rhythm with your stride. Your head wobbles on the top of this moving pyramid, adding weight to the whole process. Your brain controls all this complex motion, sending nerve signals down through the spinal cord. It takes in information from your ears, the nerves in your feet, your eyes—look, there's a bump in the sidewalk—and adjusts your plan for motion.

As you do this, you get stronger. You stimulate the body through stress; you recover, and the body strengthens. You do it again: stress, recovery, repair, strengthen. As you learn the sport, you experiment with more stress and less recovery. You build your body up so you can load it more. You learn that some kinds of background pain are good, and some are not. My general rule is that if the muscles on both sides hurt equally, I'm fine. It's a problem if, say, the right quad hurts more than the left one. Then maybe the muscle is about to tear. These distinctions are hard to discern at first, but learning to parse them is essential for training. You have to cultivate fatigue during workouts, pushing your body to the point that it hurts, but not too much. You have to live with the pain day and night when you're training hard. The body gets heavy, and there are times, deep in a marathon training cycle, when I dream of just collapsing into my bed—until I actually do and am suddenly reminded of the inflammation in my legs.

At some point, every runner goes too far. Eventually there's a hot spot in your shin or a swelling in the knee. Maybe there's a hard-to-describe ache in your iliotibial band on the outside of your knee. The injuries define and distinguish the sport. In some ways, they make it democratic. Most elite runners log about 100 to 120 miles a week, which means they're out there for about two hours a day. They know that trying to do more will lead them to the trainer's table. And so, at the very top—unlike bicycling or swimming, where you can train almost all day without injury risk—you don't get ahead by putting in more time. You get ahead by training smarter and with more focus. You get ahead by sensing the cliff before you reach the edge.

I should have learned this lesson about injuries when I was young. I didn't, but it wasn't for lack of trying. I wrecked myself on a perfectly clocked nine-month cycle: the spring of my sophomore year in high school, the winter of my junior year, the fall of my senior year, and the summer before college. Wisdom came eventually, but it came through music. In my early 20s, during my phase of obsessive guitar playing, I developed a very physical style: slapping the frets, picking hard, drumming on the body of my six-string. Eventually, the tendons in my right wrist began to ache and swell. I started icing my wrists after I practiced. Then I started taking huge doses of ibuprofen. I rekeyed my computer keyboard to the Dvorak layout, turning the key labeled "k" into the letter "t" for example, to minimize the distance my fingers had to move. I tried acupuncture, massage therapy, and steroidal injections. I began brushing my teeth with my left hand. I tried physical therapy and slept with braces on my wrists. I stopped playing concerts. For two years, I often couldn't use my right hand to open a door.

Eventually, I found myself sitting in the Union Square office of Alan Katz, an instructor of the Alexander technique, a method of posture training. Katz had asked me to bring my guitar, and he instructed me to sit down and play. I lowered my neck toward the instrument, leaned over, and began to slap the frets. I had become a showman, and I felt that putting my head next to the sound hole suggested intimacy and emotion. Almost immediately Katz began to laugh. "This won't be hard," he said.

He told me to stop playing but to keep the position. Then he walked behind me. He gently pulled my head up so that it was directly above my neck, not the fretboard. He pushed down on one arm until my shoulders were straight. He repositioned my hips and my feet so that my sit bones were directly above my heels and directly below my shoulders. My spine now ran straight from the base of the skull. My feet formed a base for my body. He had turned a crookneck squash into a broccoli stalk. Now, he said, play again.

It felt awkward, but also easier. He explained that the head weighs roughly 10 pounds. If you bend it down and over the fretboard, the muscles of the neck have to support that weight, which strains the muscles of the shoulders and then the wrists. Then he told me to stand at ease but to close my eyes. He moved my head around and adjusted my hips. He pressed on my back. He asked me how I thought I was standing. "Like a hunchback," I responded. He told me to open my eyes and look in the mirror: I was as straight as a man in the King's Guard. I just had no idea what that felt like anymore. I came back week after week, but I didn't need to. Within a month, all the pain in my wrists was gone. I could play guitar as much as I wanted. I also had begun to learn a practice that would help me prevent running injuries and heal them quickly when they came.

Running with your body completely in sync isn't easy. One of my feet is slightly larger than the other. The muscles on my left leg are larger (maybe from balancing on it while kicking soccer balls), but the muscles on my right leg work better (maybe from kicking the soccer ball). I've been warped from racing on a track, circling forever with my left shoulder tilted to the curve. I have incongruous little buckets of fat at my midsection even when I'm at my skinniest racing weight. Still, when I run, I try to keep as synchronized as possible. I think of energy flowing in a straight line between my lower back and the base of my skull. I try to land equally on the left side and the right side. When I run around Prospect Park, I alternate directions: clockwise, counterclockwise, clockwise. If no one else is on a track, I run it in reverse, with my right shoulder aimed into the curve.

Being a parent also led me to discover what I consider the ideal form of cross-training. I wrestled endlessly with my three boys. I carried them, flipped them, and played a game called "blind monster," in which they would run across mats laid around our apartment and I would try to tackle them while on my knees with my eyes closed. We played so much "hallway soccer" that we obliterated all the paint on the inside of the apartment's front door. We played Nerf basketball, where I could only block shots with my head, and we played "water wars," where I would try to swim across a pond and get up on a small beach they were guarding. Eventually, we'd play full-court basketball, but I couldn't block shots and had to let the ball bounce before I could rebound. I tried to beat them in parkour on the walks to school.

I parented this way mostly by instinct. I hadn't read a book that told me to wrestle with my kids. I just enjoyed it, and so did they. By happenstance, it kept me healthier than I've ever been in my life. I had enough cross-training to balance me and provide stability without ever causing stress. From the time Zachary first kicked a soccer ball, I have probably done some odd sport, in some odd way, every single day I wasn't traveling. I created endless chaos in our Brooklyn apartments. We broke vases, knocked over plants, and occasionally woke up the neighbors. But we had a lot of fun. And for 10 years I never once missed a workout or a race because of injury.

■

In some ways running is like farming. Our natural talent is the soil. Some of us have potential like the lush lands of the Sacramento Valley. Others are born with genes like the Siberian shrubland. Then a seed needs to drop into that soil. For my father, it happened sometime in the late 1970s, as he tried to sort out his professional and sexual identities. For me, it happened when I was cut from the high school basketball team. For others, it happens in a school sprint or when their father takes them to watch the Boston Marathon. Once in the ground, the seed needs attention, care, sunlight, and steady water. As we age into our late 20s, the soil improves. Eventually, as we pass into our 30s and 40s, the nutrients leak out of the soil and the crop starts to wilt.

One of the fundamental misunderstandings about running is that talent determines where you start and that training determines where you end. As David Epstein has explained in *The Sports Gene,* talent is also your ability to get better. In 1992, a team of researchers in the United States and Canada enlisted nearly five hundred parents and their children and put them into identical training programs. They were all scored on a metric of cardiovascular fitness called VO_2 max before the study. Then, for five months, they did the exact same stationary-cycling workouts while being measured in a lab. About 15 percent of the participants didn't improve at all, and about 15 percent significantly increased the amount of oxygen their bodies could extract from their blood. Amazingly, the amount of improvement had absolutely nothing to do with their level of fitness when they began the program. But it did seem to have something to do with genetics. "Family members generally had similar aerobic benefits from training, while variation between different families was great," Epstein wrote.

Once, I was running down Vanderbilt Avenue in Brooklyn with Julia Lucas, one of my closest running friends and a true elite. We were chatting about VO_2 max and I told her what I'd scored when it was measured in a lab. She laughed just for a second. The number was comically low for someone like her. It was as though she was a player on the Knicks meeting a new teammate who is 5'9". But she was also wise and knew that sometimes the short player has talents and gifts not immediately visible to the others. My gift, perhaps, was that I respond better to training than my peers who do the same thing. Or perhaps it's that I never got hurt, while she had struggled with injuries throughout her career. After taking a moment to compose herself, she said, "You're like a car with a tiny engine, and a chassis that never breaks. I have a huge engine and a chassis that's always cracked."

Which part, exactly, is talent?

CHAPTER 8

Julia Lucas

You don't know what got you here. It's not normal. None of this is normal. It's not normal to be this good at anything. You're only here 'cause of what's bloody wrong with you.

—MARK ROWLAND

JULIA LUCAS GREW UP IN THE PIEDMONT REGION OF CENTRAL NORTH Carolina, the flatlands between the Appalachian Mountains and the coast. Her father was an Abstract Expressionist painter. When she thinks of him back then, she sees a shirtless man flinging paint at a wall in a barn. The family was briefly homeless when Lucas was about five, living with other artists in an abandoned building in Washington, D.C. They moved to North Carolina soon after that, and she joined the school cross-country team at age 14. Lucas remembers herself as "an oblivious, happy weirdo" who started running because a friend told her everyone on the team got free Popsicles. Her parents were game; they worried about her spending too much time reading. Lucas had never done any other sports, and "cross-country" sounded mysterious. She thought that she would be running across the country, seeking out clues in the woods.

Lucas quickly discovered that she was good. In her first race, she beat all the varsity runners at her school. She remembers her coach, tabulating the scores by hand and looking at her. "Wow. Special," he exclaimed.

She wasn't a graceful runner. Having never played any other sport, she didn't have a good sense of balance. But she had an engine. She was the fastest runner in her school in every race, and soon one of the fastest runners in the state. She couldn't believe the gift she had discovered. She'd run late into the evening, with her protective father riding his bike beside her. Before races, she and a friend would holler the same lines from the movie *Gallipoli* that I had: "What are your legs?" "Springs. Steel springs." Running quickly became everything. More than the races, she remembers the feeling she had after workouts. "I'm lying on my back after a track practice. And I've got myself to some kind of oxygen depletion or weird neurological state where I'm lying on my back and my eyes are funny. The sky looks like lava. And if I don't blink, I can see everything sliding," she told me. "Getting to those physical states, just sort of a really sensual experiential zone, was entrancing."

Her legs, though, turned out not to be made of steel. In a meet during her sophomore year, she was running along in the lead when she heard a loud crack. She fell to the ground, got up, stumbled, and fell again. Her fibula had broken, and she would be in a cast for 12 weeks. She responded to her new vulnerability with obsession. She put plastic bags over her cast, duct-taped the top, and snuck into the local YMCA to run in the pool. Eventually, she came back and was fast again. As a senior, she won three North Carolina state titles.

Lucas didn't have a sense that life would happen after running. Lucas ran, ran some more, and then sat in the woods reading. She didn't pay attention in class, and she had to miss one season of track after failing math. "I didn't quite understand that a future would come and things I was doing now would help with it," she says.

Lucas starred again in college at North Carolina State, but top collegiate distance runners aren't like athletes in other sports. Lucas was one of the very best in the country, but all she got from that was a travel stipend and $15,000 a year from Reebok.

Running is the most egalitarian of sports. Anyone can put on their shoes and open the door. But as your goals become more focused, money matters. There are flights to take, trainers to pay, gear to purchase, and special meals to prepare. Lucas had Olympic goals but an overdrawn checking account. And she was now injured, having torn a muscle in her abdomen at the end of the season. One of her doctors ran his hand up her thigh and propositioned her; she pushed him away, but she had to keep coming back to him for care because she felt she had no other choice. She traveled to Portland, Oregon, to consult a movement expert, but she could afford only medical bills and not rent. She slept in Forest Park, just outside the city, and kept her belongings in a garbage bag. In the morning, she would head down to the park's concrete bathrooms to clean herself in a sink near the bottom of Wildwood Trail. Then, along with a line of other homeless people, she would walk down into the city. She hid her belongings in the woods; if it looked likely to rain, she would carry it all down to the bus station, where she could rent a locker for $2. Lucas didn't let herself think about trying something else. Like many focused athletes, she believed that when you're planning for the future, you're done with the present: "If you're sprinting with someone and they feel solid in their future and you don't, you have this something else that you can pull from. It's that totally desperate feeling: like I could die tomorrow."

Eventually, she traveled to Stockton, California, to meet Dan Pfaff, one of the gurus of the sport. He had grown up on a farm, where he studied the biomechanics of cows. He had turned that into an understanding of the biomechanics of humans. He liked Lucas's intensity and told her that he would see her for free. She came to his giant unheated warehouse, and he looked her up and down. She ran in front of him, and he put his hands on her and pushed deep into the muscle. He thought for a while and then told her what he believed to be wrong: she was missing what he called a deep core. Perhaps because she had never played sports as a child, she had no strength in a muscle called the transversus abdominis. To find it, she had to lie on her back and force her fingers under the ridge beneath her pelvis. There, she would feel a triangle between the rectus abdominus and external oblique. Pfaff told Lucas to make an image in her mind's eye of all the muscles in her abdomen. Then he said she should visualize peeling them back one by one to reach the triangle. If she focused, she could learn to isolate, flex, and strengthen it. Lucas did just that. Gradually she could run without pain. She later astonished doctors by moving this muscle precisely while they took a sonogram. They had never seen anyone else able to control it like that. One of the best things about this sport is that you can succeed just by thinking about your legs and your feet; and you can succeed, too, by thinking about cells, energy flow, and all the little muscles that most of us don't even know exist.

Lucas started getting fast again. She joined a team in Mammoth Lakes, California, but her coach was too structured and scientific. At one point, the coach had her running on a treadmill at 9,000 feet of elevation with an oxygen mask on that made her feel like she was running at sea level. After a few miles, she started sobbing. Then she ripped the mask off. "I just felt like I was the Russian from *Rocky IV*. I was just so sad, and it was so antithetical to what I thought running was."

She switched teams to the Oregon Track Club Elite with coach Mark Rowland. That was when she started to get truly good. After one meet when she had done spectacularly well, she was taking the bus back with her teammates. They were joking about her Humpty Dumpty stride and odd form. She laughed and said that she'd be a world-beater if her parents had, just once, enrolled her in some sport as a kid. She wasn't even good at tag! She was being dramatic for laughs. Coach Rowland was driving, and he slammed on the brakes and pulled the van off the highway. Lucas describes the moment in a thesis she wrote for the Iowa Writers' Workshop. "*'Don't you EVER,'* he looked back at us, over his shoulder, *'wish away what is strange about you. You don't know what got you here. It's not normal. None of this is normal. It's not normal to be this good at anything. You're only here 'cause of what's bloody wrong with you. Don't you ever let me hear you wishing you was more normal. Alright?'*"

In the spring of 2012, Lucas ran the fastest 5000-meter time of any woman in the country that year. She was at her peak and she headed to the Olympic Trials in Eugene as one of the favorites. Lucas had two ways to make the team. The easiest was to come in first, second, or third. But track rules can be strange, so she had another route as well. Because of her speedy running earlier in the season, she had what is called the Olympic standard, and many of the competitors did not. Even if she came in at the back of the pack, she could make the team if the third-place runner didn't finish faster than 15:20, the qualifying time set by the Olympics' organizers.

Lucas remembers the start of the race. The quiet. Her parents in the stands. The stadium packed. She stood at the line, windmilled her arms, rotated her ankles, and jumped. She wanted to keep the blood flowing in her body, and she wanted to quiet her mind. She looked at a family in the stands, right by the start, with two children sharing an oversized cup of frozen lemonade. "Runners on your marks," came the command. Lucas lined one toe right up to the starting line and cocked her arms. Then off they went.

The runners stayed packed together, lap after lap. Lucas's path to the Olympics was clear: they were running slower than 15:20 pace and she just needed it to stay that way. But she wanted to win outright, and she wanted to crush all the women who had gotten better contracts, gotten more attention, and never had to chase their dreams while sleeping in Forest Park. So, with three laps to go, Lucas made her move. She pulled to the front and started accelerating. The big group of runners slipped apart, like a small pile of leaves that is slowly floating down a river and then hits a waterfall. Lucas was in first, well ahead. Two other women—Molly Huddle and Julie Culley—gamely struggled to keep pace but steadily drifted back. With one lap to go, Lucas had a lead of ten meters over Huddle and Culley, and then another ten meters over the woman in fourth. I've watched the race on YouTube a dozen times, and I always think she's going to win. The camera pans as they go around the first bend and you can't even see the runner in fourth. Lucas looks smooth and strong.

But then, suddenly, she doesn't. With 300 meters to go, something goes wrong with Lucas's left leg. It looks like maybe it starts to sway a little bit to the side. Then her arms aren't in sync. Huddle and Culley approach her and then blaze by. Ten years later, Culley told me she still remembers trying to look and sound as relaxed as possible so as not to give Lucas any hope.

With 100 meters to go, Lucas is still in third, well ahead of fourth place. The camera pans back, focusing on the two leaders sprinting to the line. But in the back of the screen, you can see catastrophe. Lucas is slowing and two women are surging toward her. They approach the line. Lucas looks like an injured flamingo. Her strides have shortened and her back sways. Lucas gets to the line and her foot appears to go over first, but one of the other women, Kim Conley, is bounding from behind her like a leopard, taking one stride for Lucas's two. Conley leans forward with perfect timing. Lucas couldn't see or hear her coming. The predator always has this advantage over the prey. Conley finishes in third.

And then there's a pause. Conley didn't have the Olympic standard coming into the race. If she finished in a time slower than 15:20, it wouldn't matter what place she got. But then the scoreboard flashes:

3. KIM CONLEY   15:19.79
4. JULIA LUCAS   15:19.83.

Soon Conley is grabbing an American flag and high-fiving people in the stands. Lucas is standing alone, in tears. Then she has a microphone in her face, and she's calmly explaining how it felt and what it means. She's dripping in sweat, and the muscle on her neck bulges. She doesn't offer excuses; she just calmly explains what went wrong. When one of the reporters asks her how much it hurt, she responds, "I had no pain. No pain at all."

Years later, Lucas and I would sit and talk about the race. "I knew I had done the wrong thing, but also, I was sure that I could turn the wrong thing into the right thing," she told me. "I wanted to do something wild. I was afraid and used to bringing big, dramatic moments into times when I just didn't know what to do. When in doubt, cause chaos."

Lucas left the stadium and went home to change. Her dog, Chap, greeted her happily, wiggling around in the otherwise quiet entryway, oblivious to what had just happened. *What, you don't know?* she remembers thinking. Chap jumped and licked her, just as always. And maybe she wasn't wrong. Who has understood the moral complexities of the situation better: the humans reacting to a specific failure under arbitrarily constructed rules, or the dog who just offers blind love?

That was pretty much the end of Lucas's running career. She would stay a pro for another year, but she knew that she could never again approach the emotional intensity or the meaning of that moment. She retired, gave away all her running clothes, moved to New York, and then moved to Iowa for graduate school to become a writer.

Back in New York after school, she coached, wrote, and ran around Prospect Park. I met her at a pop-up Tracksmith store one weekend. Of course I remembered the race and the photo finish. Soon, we were running buddies, circling the park together every month or two. She seemed conflicted about the sport, but I couldn't quite figure out why. It wasn't the race; she was at peace with how that had gone.

One afternoon, we sat together at the Gold Star pub in Brooklyn with my dog, Roti. Lucas, who resembles Penelope Cruz if cast in the role of a skinny track star, fed Roti cheese and pepperoni from a plate of a nearby table's abandoned leftovers, and we talked for hours about running and her career. And then I finally came to understand the ambivalence she had about the sport and her time in it. She loved running, but she felt that she lost something in competing. One can run as a way to seek spiritual awakening, and one can run to fulfill ambition. It's often hard to do both. Trying to win had added clarity to Lucas's goals, and it had given her confidence. She had come as close as one can come to making an Olympic team, but coming so close had only made her question what she saw there. Maybe her dog had been right when she greeted Lucas so enthusiastically at the door.

I told her the story of Bobbi Gibb, running across the country with Moot, sleeping under the stars, and then heading to the next forest she could find to the west. "In my mind, that's the runner I was. But I was just too results-oriented and I wanted to beat everybody," Lucas said. She wished she had been like Gibb. "It's my dream. That should have been my way."

CHAPTER 9

Here's What's Going to Happen

Most of what I know about writing, I've learned through running every day.

—HARUKI MURAKAMI

TO RUN IN NEW ENGLAND IS TO LEARN TO APPRECIATE SEASONS, AND I feel at home in all of them. I learned at Andover to run in the dark winter mornings with socks on my hands, hopping over slush and striding through snow. I learned how to circle a track crusted in ice and how to pull back the branch of a pine tree to bring the snow down upon my teammates coming just behind. I learned how, in the crepuscular hours, to identify patches of black ice on a lonely road. In spring, there might be the scent of lilacs as I pass over the soft, wet ground, leaving faint footprints as I go. Other days, the rain comes down so hard it hurts. The lengthening days feel like they go on forever. Last year's leaves have spent months underneath snow and ice, and now they crackle as they break under my feet. Then summer comes with the fresh, cut grass and the honeysuckle. I can start a run at 4 A.M. and know there'll be light. And then autumn, with cool winds, and fresh leaves piled high on the ground. To run through the Andover bird sanctuary in October is to cross into a Winslow Homer painting. The palette changes subtly each day as the maple trees flip from green to scarlet while the oak trees stubbornly hold on to their russet leaves.

As I've become an adult, I've done most of my racing on roads. I like big-city marathons with precise courses lined by Porta-Potties. I set a goal, adjust it for the weather, and then track my miles to the second. I like the camaraderie of crowded start lines as a C-level celebrity sings the national anthem. I like the finish lines, where runners stumble around in space blankets looking like Rodin statues—their bodies strong and sinewy, their faces haggard and drawn. I like races where you aren't really racing anyone in particular, but everyone is racing the same clock. Still, when I dream about running, it is these early sensory memories that come back. I see mountains, narrow pine-needle paths, and birch trees. I fell in love with the sport on Holt Hill, on Kinsman, on the Around Mountain loop in Maine. I fell in love with the sport when I learned to push myself slowly upward in the style of a mountain runner—stride shortening, forefoot hitting the ground first, my heel never quite touching down—until I could make it up to the tree line.

In the summer of 2012, I entered an 18-mile race, the Escarpment Trail Run, through the Catskills. Mountain running requires a particular kind of strength and a particular kind of balance, but I couldn't train properly for it. I live in Brooklyn, where the roads are paved and the wildest animals are the rats. So, I improvised. While commuting in through Manhattan, I'd hurdle crates of mushrooms outside bodegas or try to run on the narrow edges of sidewalks to improve my coordination. I'd step over the white lines in crosswalks, turning them into mini-agility ladders. I'd try to improve my peripheral vision by staring straight ahead and working to read the street signs on either side of me. I'd run-commute to a collection of boulders down at South Cove by Battery Park City and jump from rock to rock with my commuting backpack on. As I ran up the steps to the Brooklyn Bridge, I'd push aside the dank stench of urine and imagine I was bounding on a Catskills trail. Then, one Sunday in July, in a ritual I'd continue most Julys for eight years, I'd wake up at 5 A.M. and drive north to the start.

The Escarpment Trail Run begins in a parking lot, but you quickly file onto a narrow, wooded path that climbs for three straight miles up Windham High Peak. You follow the colored blazes on the trees, twisting over the roots and ducking under branches. The path is gnarled and never straight: run around a corner too fast and you'll crash into a tree. Scamper too quickly up a rocky outcrop and your foot will slip on wet, slimy moss and you'll go tumbling back down. You have to worry about bears, snakes, and hornets. Approaching a peak, you pass a white single-engine airplane that crashed near the course during a foggy morning in 1983. Once you reach the top, unfortunately, you have to go down. Descending a mountain is like skiing: speed is determined by experience and skill more than fitness. You go fast when you're not afraid to fall. I progress with the brakes on, grabbing trees for balance, stopping, looking over ledges. My peers bomb downward, jumping off ledges, landing with one foot on a slippery rock and then launching to the next one. They run like they're in free fall, using their feet like hooves, and they pass me like horses racing past a cow. The greatest mountain runner in the world, Kilian Jornet, sometimes trains by memorizing terrain and then running with his eyes closed. He attributes his skill partly to a childhood in the Spanish Pyrenees in which his mother would take him out into the woods in his pajamas at night and have him lead the way home in the darkness. He can bend his ankle sideways and jump up and down landing on it. Running downhill, he says, is like dancing. I've never been a good dancer, and my mother never took me into the woods in my pajamas, so I struggle on the descents. But down I would go on the trails through the lovely Catskills mud. Then up. Then down. Then up. Finally, I would sprint along a ledge, trying not to tumble hundreds of feet off the side, and cross the finish line. That's where I would stop, breathe, and bless the heavens that I was alive to do this. "Live in the sunshine, swim in the sea, drink the wild air," Ralph Waldo Emerson once wrote.

I finished the race several times with blood coming from my knees, and once from my shoulder. Other runners finished with concussions and busted ankles. They would cross the line hobbled, but not quite looking as wan as the runners near me in my other races. Mountain runners are built more like soccer players than like elite marathoners. Their bodies need to be optimized for balance, agility, and fuel storage. One year, Danielle came to the finish and declared that the top finishers "look much more normal than the people who usually beat you."

■

Nine months after my first Escarpment race, I was in my office at *The New Yorker,* tracking the Boston Marathon, the oldest marathon in the world. I grew up near the 21-mile marker of the course, and I cherish early memories of the race. The first sporting event I remember watching was the famous battle in the 1982 race between Alberto Salazar and Dick Beardsley. Salazar wore red shorts and propelled himself forward awkwardly, somehow combining the speed and power of Achilles with the clumsy cadence of a man hustling to the restroom. They ran so close together that Beardsley monitored Salazar by watching his shadow.

This year, in 2013, I tracked my friends, all of whom finished smoothly. Then news alerts started popping up on my phone. Something had exploded on the marathon course. Could it have been an accident? No. Someone had set off a bomb on the north side of Boylston Street, just before the finish line. I watched in horror as men and women covered in blood ran away from the place everyone had just been running toward.

I had by then moved from editing print features to managing *The New Yorker*'s website. My boss, David Remnick, appeared at the door of my office. He told me that I was the person on staff who had to write about this. I was a runner, after all. I protested: I had writers to edit and editors to manage. I didn't say it out loud, but I had much more confidence in others to write about this than I had in myself. Remnick had started as a newspaper reporter and once had bylines on the front page of *The Washington Post* for eight consecutive days. He is one of the people I respect most in the world, but patience is not his greatest virtue. "Here's what's going to happen," he said. "You're going to close the door after I leave and turn off your phone. I'm going to come back in an hour, and you're going to give me your piece."

I started to write. When a man knows he is to be hanged in a fortnight, it concentrates his mind wonderfully. One hour

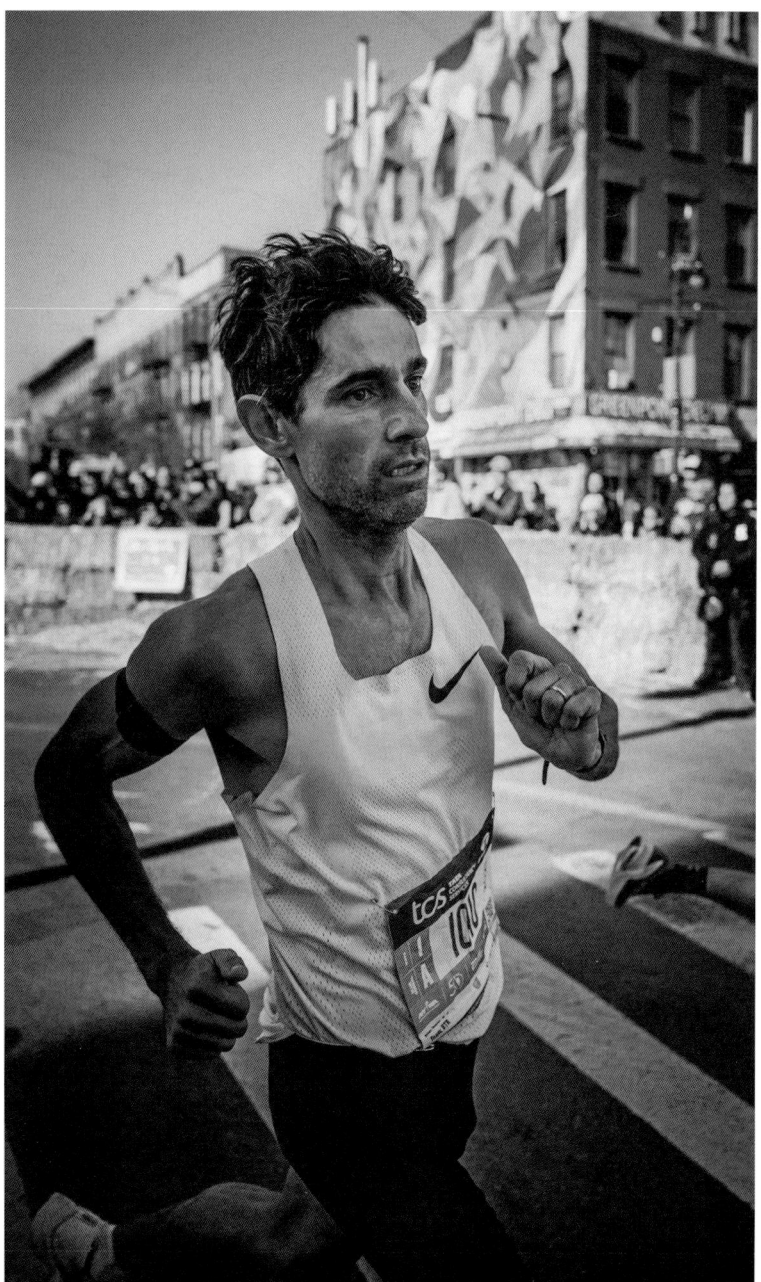

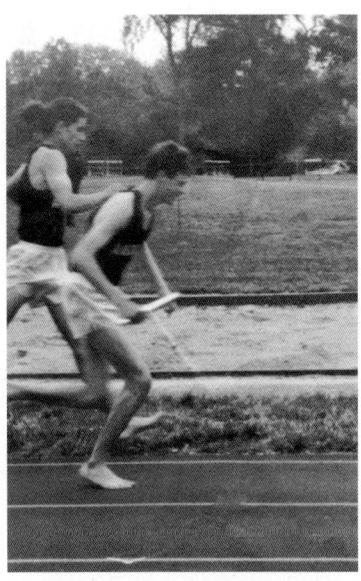

Me in ponytail, with Tim Roberts, running a barefoot relay race for Andover, 1993.

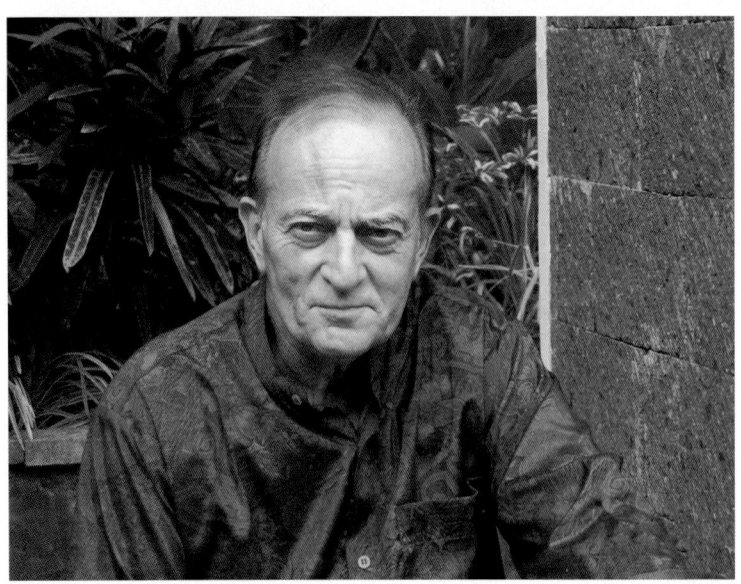

Scott Thompson, Bali, 2004.

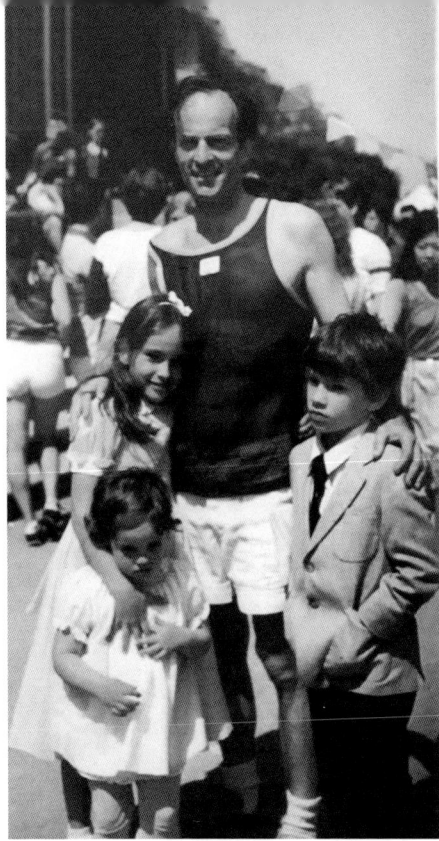

After a race, and church for the kids, around 1981.

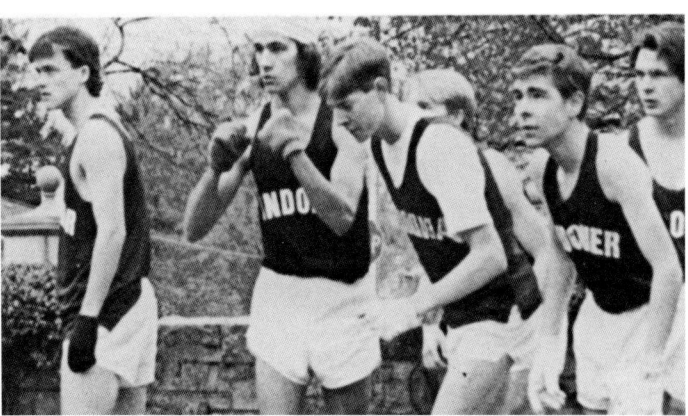

Me in gloves, fall of 1992 at Andover.

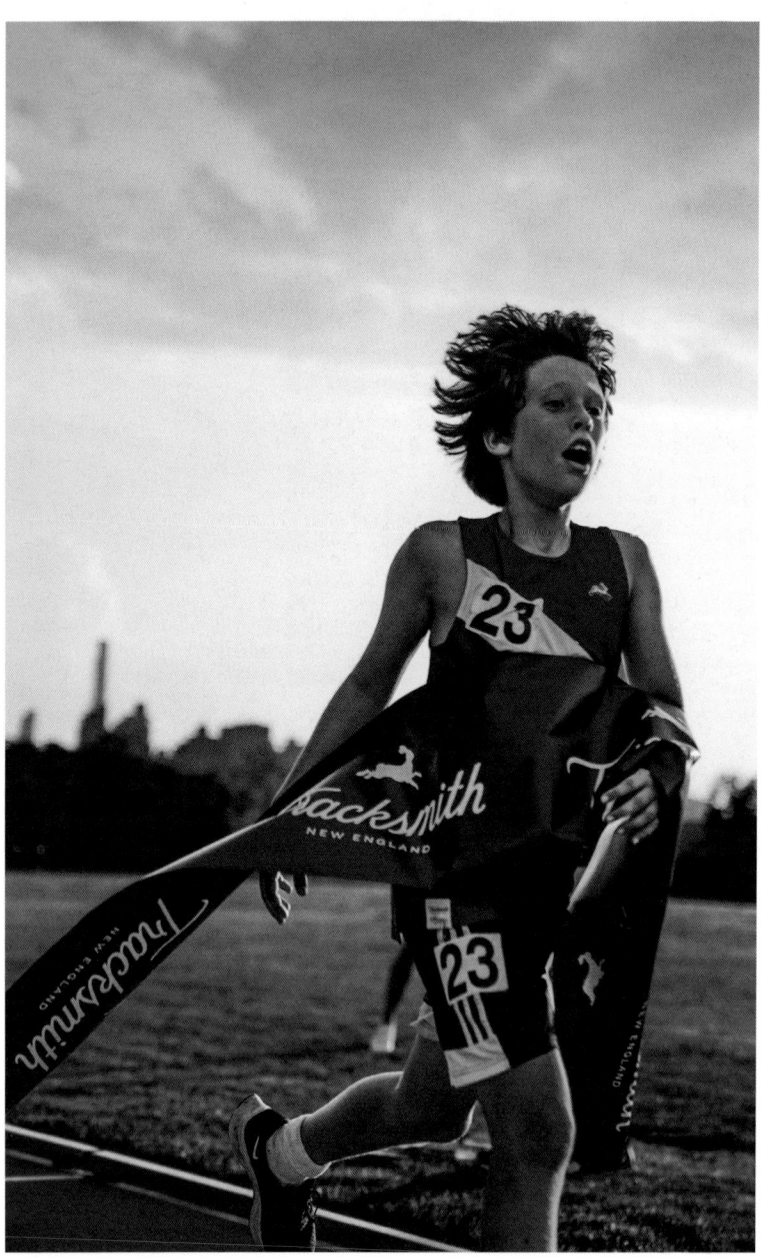
Zachary winning a 5K in New York City, 2021.

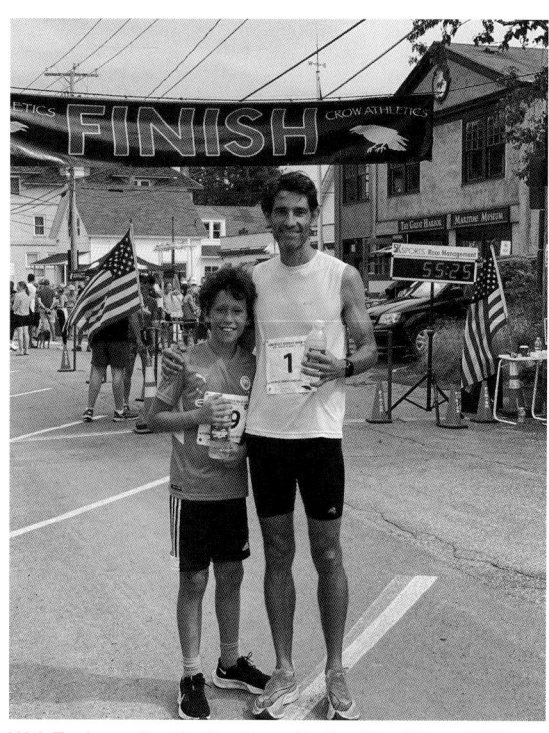

With Zachary after the Northeast Harbor Road Race, 2021.

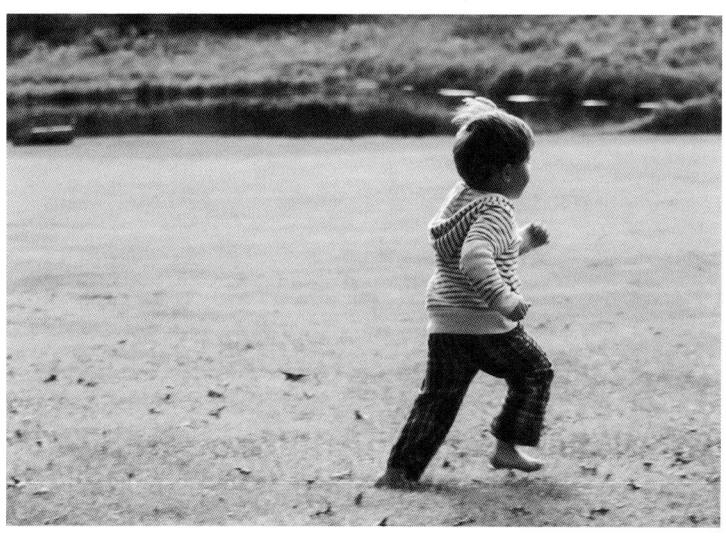

Ellis, around 2010.

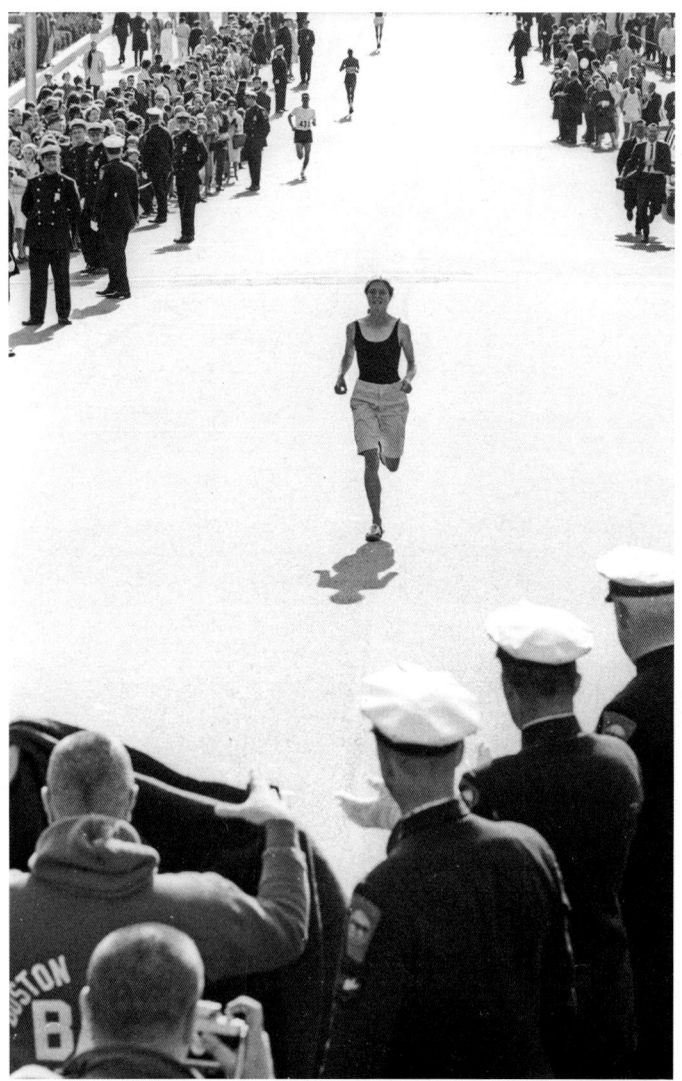

Bobbi Gibb at the end of the 1966 Boston Marathon.

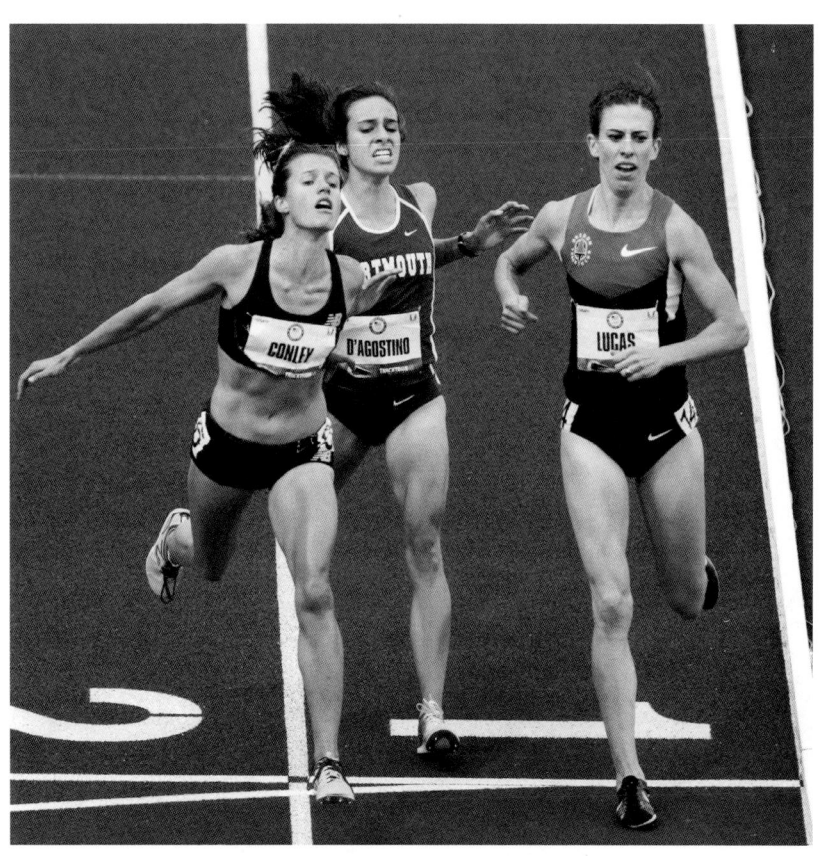

From left to right: Kim Conley, Abbey D'Agostino, and Julia Lucas, during the women's 5000-meter final at the 2012 U.S. Olympic Trials.

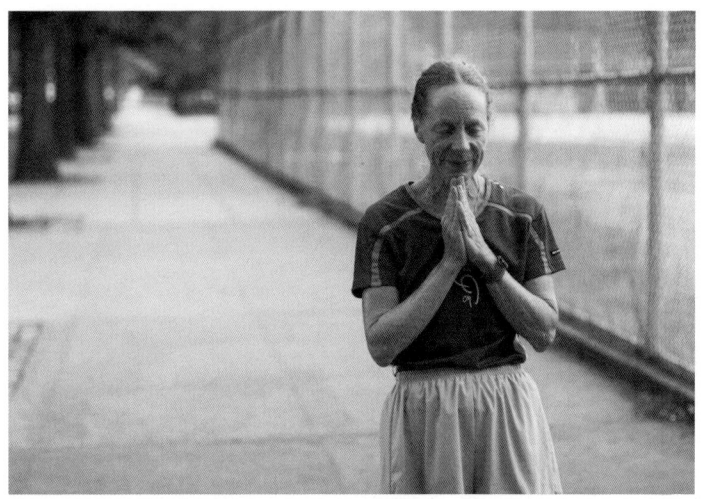

Suprabha Beckjord on day 57 at the 2008 Sri Chinmoy Marathon.

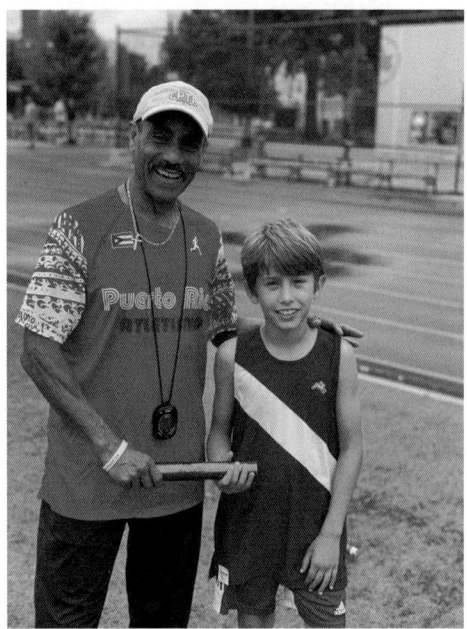

Tony Ruiz and James.

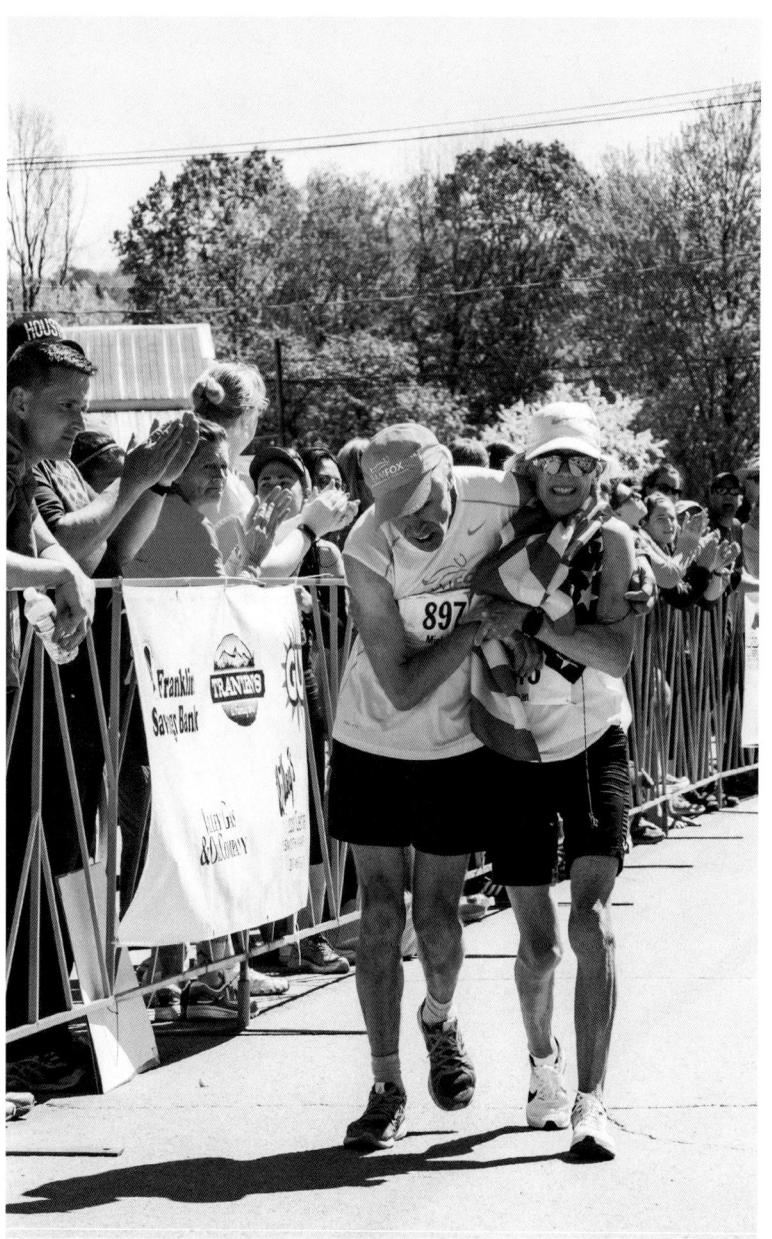

Michael Westphal, left, at the finish of the 2017 Sugarloaf Marathon in Kingfield, Maine.

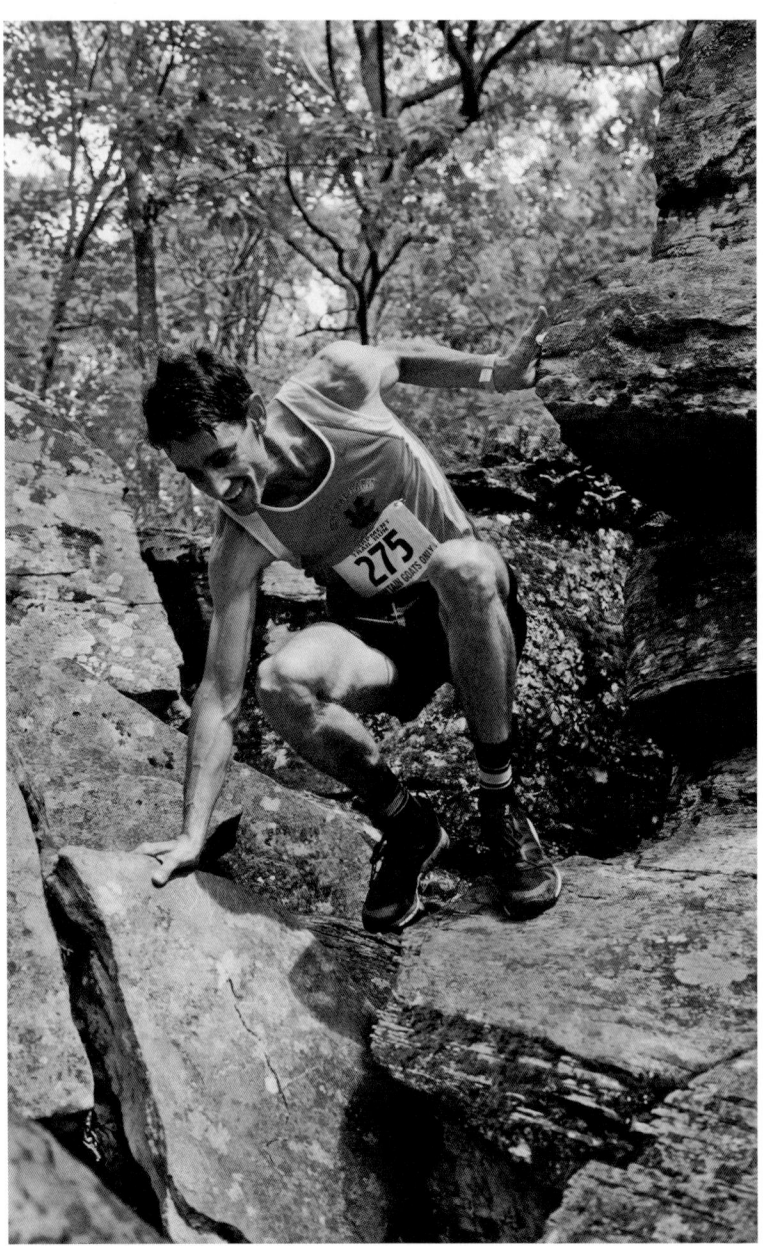

Escarpment Trail Run, 2018.

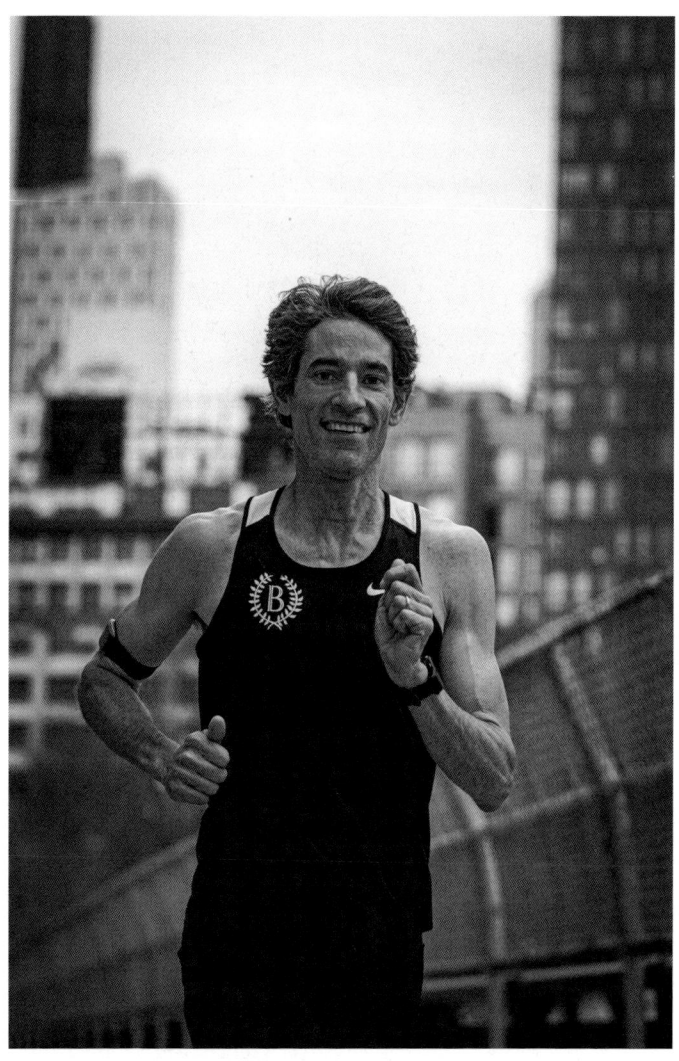

On the Manhattan Bridge during the East River Ekiden 50K, 2025.

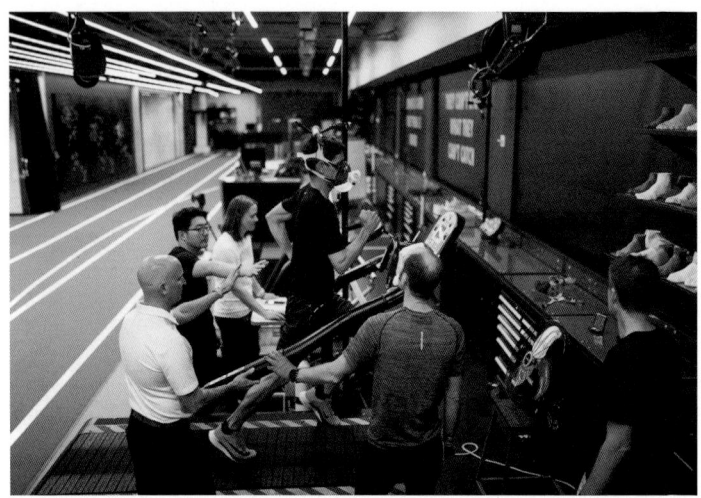

In the Nike lab, 2018.

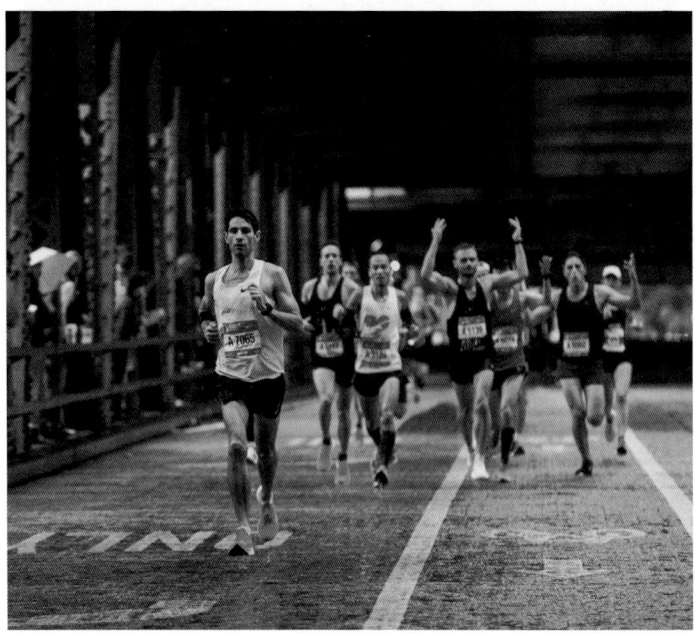

Chicago Marathon, 2018.

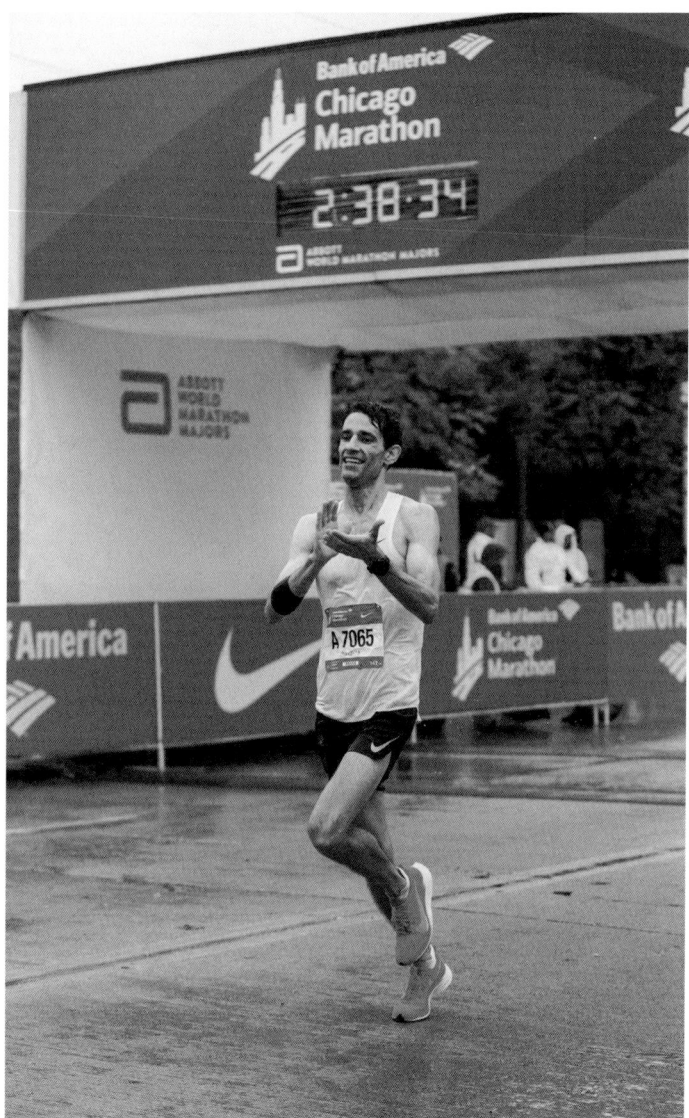

Chicago Marathon, 2018.

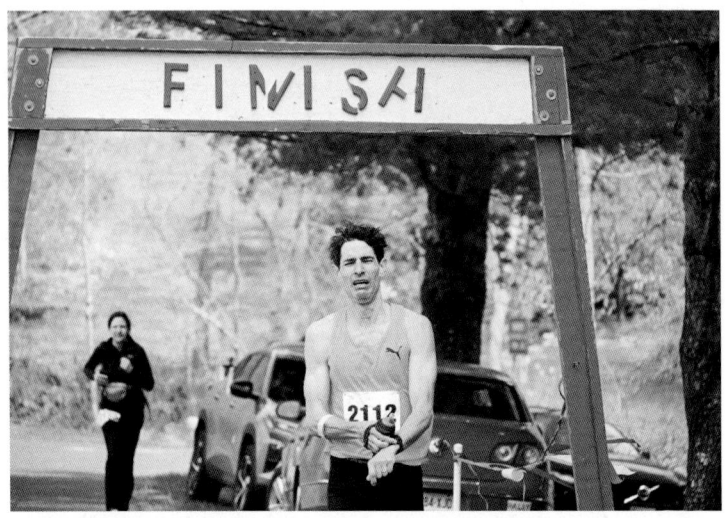

Finishing the 2025 Jack Bristol 50-miler.

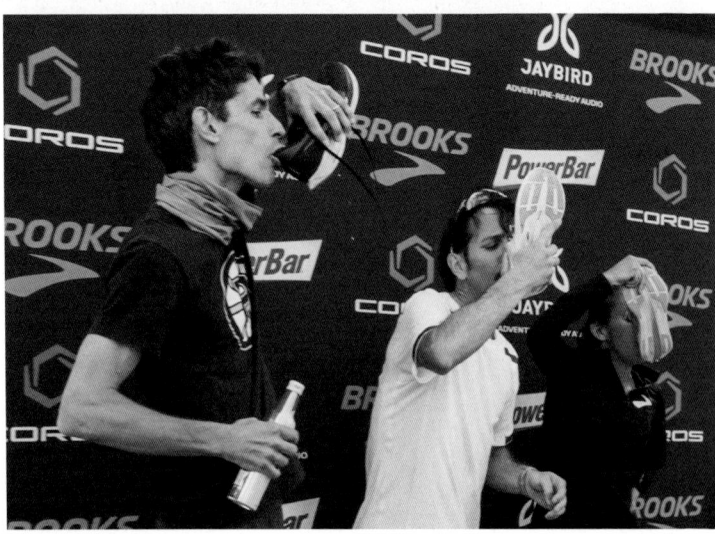

After setting the 50K record in 2021, with Desiree and Ryan Linden.

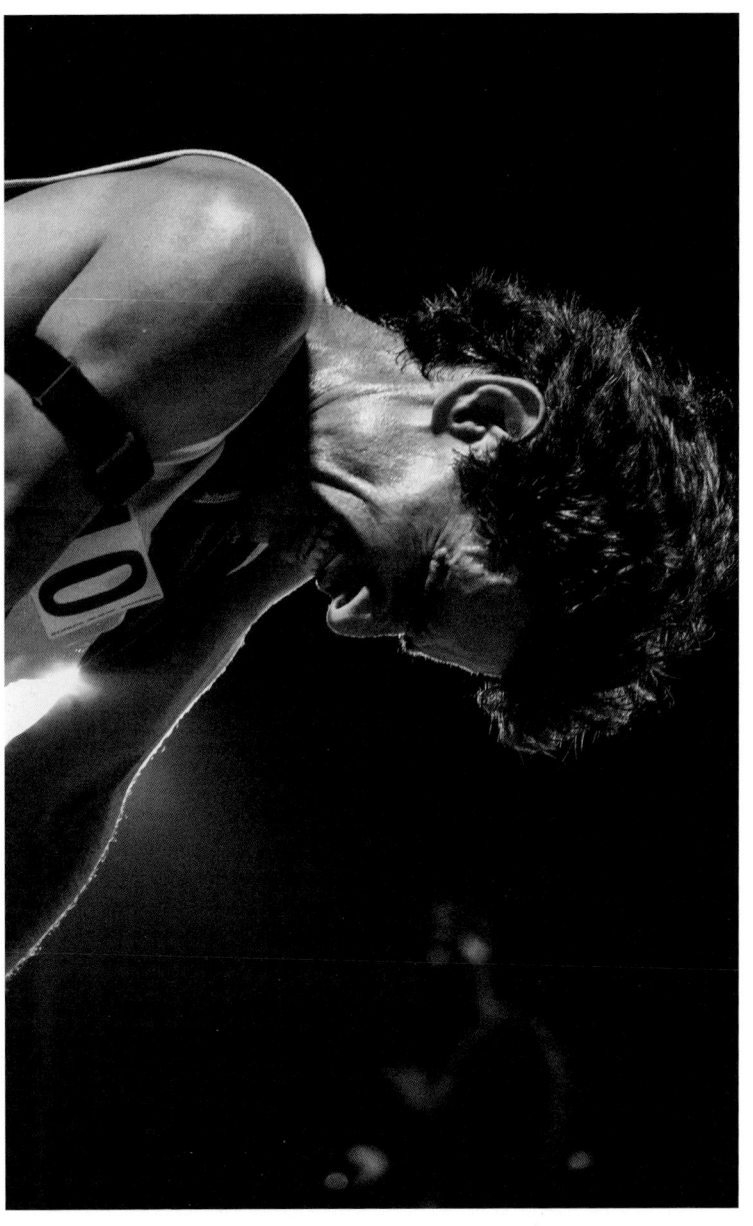

After a 5K in New York City, 2021.

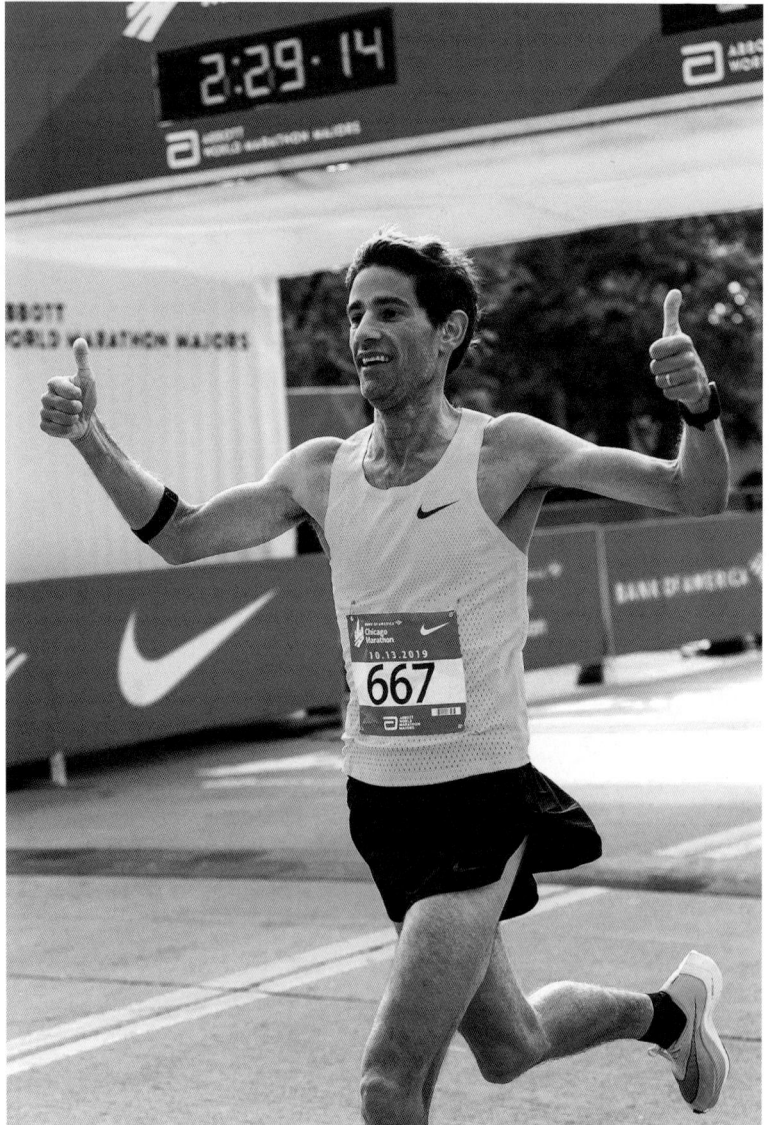

later, Remnick arrived as promised, and I handed him a piece. "The end of the marathon is where one thinks, also, about what a person, and a body, can take—human endurance. The switch to contemplating its vulnerability was sudden and abrupt," I wrote. A few hours later, I published a second story along with a photograph from Getty of a woman walking backward against the crowd of runners who didn't yet know the race had ended. She had short hair, tied tightly back, and her sunglasses were up on her head. Her hands were folded in a triangle up against her mouth. The caption read, "a woman near Kenmore Square." Remnick had taught me a lesson about writing that matched one I had already learned about running: the best time to do something important is usually right now. And when you have to "get something done quickly," it's wise not to spend that time complaining about how little time you have.

The next day, I got an email from a woman named Emily Locher. "The cover photo of your 'meaning of Boston Marathon' story is me. I had been stopped by race officials and was walking back along the course trying to find a friend I thought was behind me. Feel free to contact me if you want more info. My fourth Boston—on such a perfect day meant to celebrate achievement and life, for such a tragedy."

I called her, and she told me her story. She lived in Weston, Connecticut, with her husband and was a lawyer at an asset-management company. She ran her first marathon in 1998, and she first met the qualifying standards for Boston in 2004. The fastest she had ever run a marathon was 3:36. This year, though, she wasn't really thinking about time. "I was diagnosed with breast cancer about eighteen months ago," she told me. "Toeing the line was the big deal for me." She had had an elective double mastectomy and extensive chemotherapy. But she had tried to train throughout. Every day she went in for treatment, she made sure to run. Maybe it was just a mile or two, and maybe it was slow. But it meant something to do something.

Suddenly, near the very end of the race, she was told to stop. She hadn't heard the explosions, and she didn't know what was going on. But then she started to hear about the horror from people on the sidelines. She and the other runners waited in a crowd, with more runners filing in, like cars slowing to a halt on a highway where there's been a crash. Soon, she turned around and started to walk backward, looking for a friend with whom she had started the race. She was starting to get cold, which, she says, may be why her hands were at her face. "I was nervous and hopeful," she told me.

The bombs killed three people and injured around 300. I edited story after story tracking the hunt for the killers with a journalistic energy and anger I'd never felt before. This was my country, my city, my sport. It was also, I was coming to realize, the moment where the website I ran finally started to matter. Newyorker.com had long been the beleaguered outpost of the magazine. It was like we were the Minsk desk for a company that had a thriving office in Paris. I would hire people to work on the web by promising that I'd help them try eventually to work for the print magazine. Now, though, everyone was reading us and talking about us. Famous staff writers who had rejected our pleas in past months were sending us copy. It was better to write about a story that changed by the hour for a website than for a print magazine that came out once a week. Now we were like Abu Dhabi after the discovery of oil. The great novelist Haruki Murakami sent in an essay: "For me, it's through running, running every single day, that I grieve for those whose lives were lost and for those who were injured on Boylston Street."

Four days after the attack, one of the two terrorists, who were brothers, was dead, and the other was captured while hiding in a boat behind a house in the suburb of Watertown. The surviving murderer, Dzhokhar Tsarnaev, had written on the vessel's walls that the brothers were trying to exact revenge against the U.S. government for killing innocent Muslims. He and his brother had picked the Boston Marathon because it was indeed a symbol of hope and freedom. It was also what experts called a soft target. It had been easy for the brothers to slip in, wearing baseball caps, among the fans. The second bomb killed an eight-year-old boy who had just gotten ice cream.

■

Shortly after the Boston Marathon bombings, my dad sent me an email about *The New Yorker*'s coverage. He told me to frame our Boston Marathon stories before he abruptly switched to the topic of his now-battered farm in Warrenton, Virginia. He hadn't sold it when he moved to Asia because he thought he might want to come back. Now he was worried about it. He wanted me to write to the electric company to get the power turned back on, even though he was several years behind on the bill. He wanted me to clear it out and get it inspected. His hope was to sell the farm to an upwardly mobile Virginia family, but it looked like the setting of *The Blair Witch Project*.

My father had been neglecting the house for years. When he'd lived in Washington years before, he would leave our two

Irish setters alone at the Virginia house all week, with the doggy door open and big bowls of food outside. Whenever we arrived there, the dogs would hear the car rumbling down the driveway and race out, leaping up on us with paws flying toward our faces in a blur of reddish fur. They looked none the worse, except they would be covered in dozens of ticks, some the size of grapes, which my sisters and I would pluck out and stomp. They'd also customized the interior of the house to their liking: after sitting on the couch, you'd have to find masking tape to remove their fur from your clothes.

Dad cut corners on everything. If the roof had a leak, he would hire a day laborer off the street in nearby Manassas and then boast about how much money he had saved instead of calling a roofer. He had once dated an interior decorator who convinced him to paint the swimming pool black. The unfortunate side effect was that animals didn't realize it was there, and we were constantly fishing out dead rabbits. My sister Phyllis once had the unfortunate task of extracting a long-deceased Rottweiler.

Now it had been two years or so since anyone had swept the floor. When I traveled down to check on the house, one of the windows was broken, and I found a full bird's nest inside the living room. The basement had flooded with two feet of water. The ceiling had come down in places. There were so many dead bugs in the windows that I just opened the screens and swept them out with a broom. The couches had been chewed through by something or someone. The swimming pool, cluttered with animal corpses, would have fit a scene in a Stephen King novel. Years before, my father had planted bamboo by the porch, overlooking the pool; it was, he said, a plant that was both strong and flexible, which is how one should be in life. The bamboo was both of these things, but it was also invasive, and it had engulfed the entire back of the house. I would have needed a family of ravenous pandas to clear a path to the back door.

I did my best to help. I tried to fix the window and I removed the nest without asking the birds for back rent. I convinced the electric company to turn the power back on, and I got an inspector to come. Unfortunately, he left less than ten minutes after arriving. He almost knocked over a bee's nest at one of the doors, declared that the house smelled terrible and was probably unsafe, and then fled.

After he left, I walked down to the old swimming hole. The field we'd crossed to get there was now a forest, but you could still discern the outlines of the path we had worn 25 years before. There was an abandoned trailer at the top of the hill, left there by a handyman to whom my father had traded an acre of land for work that was never done. I wandered down to the stream, pushing bushes out of the way. The creek still ran, and our dam had long ago washed away. If you looked closely, however, you could see an unusual number of rocks piled in that part of the stream. The water, I thought, still flowed just a little bit faster there.

I did find one thing of value: a file cabinet sitting out in front of the house, barely sheltered from the wind and rain. One drawer housed a snake, but the next contained a pile of papers. I dumped out the snake, shoved the cabinet into my car, and drove it back to New York. My dad said he didn't know what the papers were and didn't want them shipped, so I stored them away and didn't look at them for years. When I finally decided to sort them out, I found, buried in old bank statements and worthless receipts, my father's diaries.

■

On a Friday night in December 2016, I sat in a corner of my Brooklyn apartment trying to sort out a conundrum. Danielle, the three boys, and I lived right off Prospect Park. Our sixth-floor apartment jutted out in a triangle toward Grand Army Plaza. I was settled in a purple wingback chair between bookcases and my guitars. A photograph of my father running in the early 1980s was on the wall above me.

I loved my job editing *The New Yorker* website. But I had been simultaneously offered two astonishing new opportunities. The major tech platforms were coping with the chaos that followed the 2016 election, and they wanted people with experience in both tech and media to help figure out what to do. One of them had offered me a great job. Meanwhile, David Remnick had put me forward as the next editor in chief of *Wired*, a sister publication under our parent company, Condé Nast.

I couldn't talk to anyone about the jobs, and I had to choose quickly. I made lists of the opportunities and risks. What was the best thing that could happen and what was the worst? Where would I be in one year, five years, ten years? Which could have more societal value? I worried about media's economic decline; I worried about getting lost in a big tech company. Danielle would talk with me, interrogate my arguments, leave, and then go read in the living room. She wasn't trying to push me one way or the other; she just wanted to guide me deeper into questions where I felt stuck. I would wander down the hallway, past the small room where two-year-old James was sleeping and the room where Ellis and Zachary, then eight and six, were bunked. Danielle and I would chat, and then I would return to my lair. She held her hands together like a quivering arrow and joked that she was keeping a probability needle, as *The New York Times* had done in the recent election.

I hadn't made up my mind by Saturday, and we went about our day. In the afternoon, I asked Zachary and Ellis to come run a mile with me in Prospect Park. Running wasn't something I did much with them, and when I did it was almost never with both together. Running at a relaxed and easy pace with your brother is no easy skill to learn. But they were game. We laced and Velcroed up and jogged toward Grand Army Plaza as a pack of three. Zachary was wearing a thin blue coat, and Ellis, who follows sports only when they provide an excuse for European travel, was wearing an FC Barcelona jersey.

Nothing makes me more worried about failure than parenting. Was I pushing the kids too much? Bones are frail at that age, and psyches are too. Were they intrinsically motivated to do this, or were they just doing it to please me? We turned around at the crest by the water fountain and made it an even mile. We stopped for apple cider doughnuts at the farmers market and then walked home, faces flushed.

That evening, after telling them bedtime stories and playing guitar for James, I dropped into my purple chair. I started to go through my lists again. Should I add weights and scores to different variables? Should I just flip a coin and try to decide, while it was in the air, what side I was rooting for? I went to complain to Danielle. "What if," she suggested, "you don't try to decide on all the things, but you just try to decide on one thing?"

This made sense. I would select a single, singularly important variable and then choose entirely based on that. After my run that evening, it seemed easy: What choice would make me a better father for my kids? I would discard all the other variables. Danielle agreed. She works as hard at her job as I work at mine, but her most important role is as a mother and mine is as a father. We should decide based on this.

Now I'd simplified it. Working in Silicon Valley would be a challenge, but I'd be entering a world that Ellis, Zachary, and James wouldn't understand at all. I'd be fussing with algorithms and partnerships. At *Wired*, I'd be testing gadgets, assigning stories, and reporting. I'd have to work all the time, but it would make more sense to them at this age. I said yes to *Wired* and became the publication's fifth editor in chief.

CHAPTER 10

Saying Thanks in the Twilight Zone

ME: What's the run you enjoyed the most?
ZACHARY, AGE 14: I enjoyed the workouts we did before the big tryout when I was nine. I remember it was raining and we were doing hill sprints in Prospect Park. I felt really motivated. It's less important where you are, and it's more important how motivated you are.

MANY THINGS DROVE MY FATHER TO MADNESS IN HIS FINAL YEARS. BUT as I came to understand his life better, I realized that nothing marked him more deeply than the death of his friend Roger Hansen, also known as "Denny."

Hansen was in some ways my father's twin. He had grown up in California, gone to Yale, and won a Rhodes Scholarship six years before my father did. Alfred Eisenstaedt had photographed Hansen's college graduation from Yale for *Life* magazine. Later that year, the magazine had published a second article on him. "It was probably the original *Life* piece that made Denny a symbol of achievement and promise," wrote Calvin Trillin in his biography of Hansen, *Remembering Denny*. "But when I try to describe what was special about him, I go from the *Life* piece to the smile. The smile was one reason he didn't seem like someone in Phi Beta Kappa. It was the smile of a candidate—someone who hired Phi Beta Kappas to do his position papers."

Like my father, Hansen's peers assumed he would become president or at least secretary of state. But life wasn't easy for Hansen when he came back from Oxford. Rhodes Scholarships are useful, but they are not amulets. Hansen was rejected from the Foreign Service, perhaps, he surmised, because he was beginning to grapple with depression and was seeing a psychoanalyst. He struggled through jobs in the television industry. He joined the Carter Administration but didn't last long. Eventually, he went into academia. His friends were nonplussed when they realized he was managing tense relations with the political science department rather than with the Republic of China. Like my father, his greatest professional achievements happened before he turned 40, or perhaps 25. Like my father, he ran. And like my father, he was gay.

These were trying years for gay men to come of age in. In his book, Trillin wrote, "Emerging from college in 1957 may have been good timing in any number of ways, but for those among us who were gay, it seems to me, the timing could hardly have been worse." If Hansen had been 20 years older, he would have just stayed in the closet. If he had been 20 years younger, he would have come out. Instead, he grappled with his sexuality in the shadows, spending time at gay bars at the edge of town and withdrawing from his straight friends. He and my father connected in the 1980s and bonded over their shared journey and struggles.

Hansen suffered from severe depression, and he leaned on my father for help. In the winter of 1990, Hansen asked to borrow my father's house in Rehoboth Beach, Delaware, a town with a thriving gay community about two and a half hours east of Washington, where the men had spent many happy days together. Now Hansen was suffering from severe back problems and he could no longer exercise. My father thought it would be a useful retreat for his friend and a chance to reset over a weekend.

On the following Tuesday, though, Hansen's psychiatrist reported that Hansen had missed a session for the first time. After my father was unable to get hold of him, a police officer broke into the garage of my father's house. Hansen had put a book and a frying pan on the gas pedal of his Honda, turned the key in the ignition, and then gone back inside to take sleeping pills. He had padded the car with pillows from my father's bedroom, perhaps intending to give himself a comfortable ending place. But he had taken so many pills, and filled the garage so densely with carbon monoxide, that he just collapsed to the cement floor and died there.

Hansen's suicide left a wound in my father's mind that never healed. It's hard to lose a friend; it's harder to lose someone you think of as a twin; it's harder still if it happens in your own garage; and it's even worse if you can't drop the thought that it could have, or should have, been you. My father would obsess about Hansen's death for the rest of his life. He wondered what else he could have done, and he wondered what else Hansen could have done. He believed that Hansen had been too closeted, too focused on keeping up appearances, too uptight. And it was from this moment on that my father decided to do the opposite. He would be flamboyant and open.

In later years, my father would often measure his own struggles against Hansen's, as if trying to calculate his distance from the abyss. He once sent me an email comparing his depression to his old friend's.

> I don't think parents should burden children with their difficulties (though I know I have, and I regret it) but I think children should know when there is a diagnosed illness which is highly treatable and remediable, especially with the understanding of those around him who love and care about him. . . . My form of depression is relatively mild, maybe 3 on a scale of 10 where Roger Hansen . . . reached 9 or 10, and I don't see any reason why it should get worse. I think it weaves in and out of my life. . . . The real point is that I think I now see how it hits and I think I see the rocks along the wall of the deep well that one falls into.

■

When my father moved to Asia, things were not going well. He had lost money on real estate trades, a gardening business, and most of his investments. He probably ended up in court with two-thirds of the people he ever did a deal with. I'm convinced that he burned down a guest house at the farm in Virginia for the insurance money, though he always blamed it on disgruntled former tenants. He was over-leveraged in everything: financially and emotionally. He was, in many ways, running aground.

He had an academic interest in Southeast Asia, as well as a particular affinity for a part of the world that helped him avoid American taxes and have more sex. He had fallen behind on the former and was addicted to the latter. Sex was his absolute obsession in later life. He once told a friend that he couldn't sleep unless he had five orgasms a day, and I don't doubt it. He once told my sister Phyllis that he hadn't spent a night alone in 20 years. His hard drive was filled with half-written novels about genuinely perverse fantasies. Phyllis once opened the door of a closet in my father's house, and an array of different-sized dildos came tumbling down on her. My younger sister, Heidi, at about age eight, put the videocassette from a *West Side Story* box in the player only to discover, to her immense confusion, that the video inside was a porn film.

He was drawn to a particular type of young man: lean, angular, and reserved. He knew that the relationships were transactional, but he was happy with his side of the deal. As a nearly bankrupt expat pretending to be rich, he bought a share of a place to live in the Philippines and leased a plot of land in Bali, where he built a villa and staffed it with men he had found online. Of his dozens, possibly hundreds, of boyfriends in a given year, some robbed him, and some told him that they loved him. Some remained at the villa in Bali, where they provided sexual services to American guests. When people asked me what my parents did for a living, I would generally answer, "My mother is an art historian and my father runs a male brothel in Bali." I would try to say it as matter-of-factly as I could, hoping to catch the listener off-guard. My father noted this line in his diaries and added that it was not unfair.

At least once a year, he would send me a note about having found a new soulmate somewhere, but I can recall only a small fraction of the names of the 20-year-old men he had told me at one point or another would be his partner for life: Bright, Ricky, Romulo, Naveen, Noriel, Ross, Jazz, Jojo, Don, Miguel, Kevin, Jon-Jon, and then another Jon-Jon. At his house in Washington, he once introduced me and Danielle to a new boyfriend, who looked just like the last boyfriend. My father put his arm around him and explained that they were going to be together forever. They were sitting on a charmingly upholstered eighteenth-century French settee, which was otherwise covered in unopened mail from Bank of America. He said they would soon be exchanging rings. I gave the union my best wishes, and then headed to the kitchen to get a glass of water. Danielle was new to this routine. She followed me into the kitchen and asked in a hushed, and worried, voice, "Isn't this really important?" I shook my head and told her it wouldn't last a week, which of course it didn't.

I wished he would settle down, and I was delighted when, in 2007, he traveled to Massachusetts to marry a young Filipino man named Louie, who I genuinely liked. But the marriage wasn't close to monogamous. My father's age plus that of his current boyfriend's always roughly equaled 80, which was fine when he was 50 and less good when he was 60. As he got into his 70s, he didn't seem able to hold a conversation for more than half an hour without bringing up what an active sex life he still had. It wasn't only that he liked to keep people off-balance. He seemed to think that the fellows he met on Yahoo! Messenger would keep him young.

One day, several months after my father had returned to Asia after a trip to Washington, I logged on to the library computer at the Metropolitan Club in Washington, a private club for the city's elite. I was immediately greeted by a photograph of a shirtless young man and the message "Hello Scotty!" It turned out my father had been surfing gay hookup sites on the same computer and had neglected to log out of Yahoo! Messenger. All the congressmen and lobbyists who'd used the computer since had apparently not known how to change it. I hurriedly found the button to log him out. I wrote to him about what happened, and he shrugged it off. It might have done the members some good, he said.

More so than with anyone else I've ever met, as the saying goes, the love that dare not speak its name had become the love that would not shut up. I was delighted that he had told many of the men at the Metropolitan Club that he was gay. I didn't think they needed access to his Yahoo! Messenger account. My father was clearly an addict, and he was clearly oblivious. I feared that to some degree he recounted his sexual conquests because he had few professional ones to describe.

I often heard him tell his boyfriends about the marathons he had run many years back. It made him seem vital. Sometimes they were intrigued, and the two of them would head out the door together for a run. So this was probably the way he ran the last time: run-shuffling on a narrow road in Bali by the rice paddies, or near the hill overlooking the village where he lived in the Philippines with some guy he'd met on Manhunt.com. I picture him wearing a short-sleeved polo shirt that he'd bought from a street merchant somewhere. He sweat a lot, and he probably didn't go far. When he got back, he probably had a glass of orange juice with seltzer.

Sometimes my father would say that he expected to live to 100. He was so similar, he thought, to his grandmother Long who had died at 99 years and 364 days. Other times, he would tell me the end was near and that he had to pass on information about his will, which he was too disorganized to assemble. I wanted him to move back to the United States, where there was better healthcare and phone service that worked all the time. But I didn't have a chance. His past accomplishments no longer mattered back home, and he owed too many people money. He felt that the country had rejected him, so he had rejected it in turn. The only time I was glad he lived abroad was when debt collectors called me trying to track him down.

With each new financial calamity, he would decamp to an ever poorer region so that he could still try to live as he had in his former life. By the end, he was in the Philippines, near a lake in Batangas Province, where some of the men called him "Sir Scott." He wrote in his unpublished memoir, "My daily life was a small court, where I could pretend to be Arthur at the Round Table." I told him I was scared that he would have some medical disaster and wouldn't be able to get to a hospital. He told me not to worry.

■

My father knew that his biggest health risk was a heart attack. His father had died of one. His grandfather had too. But he would always claim that his years of marathoning offered him protection. He wasn't wrong; running is a way to counter that particular genetic curse, even as the alcohol, stress, cigarettes, and so much else in his life worked in the other direction. He wrote once, "Marathons, even if they wore down my hips, continue to minimize the usual form of death in my family history—heart failure."

It's unquestionably the case that running regularly is better for one's health than not running at all. Study after study has shown that aerobic exercise reduces the risk of all cardiovascular diseases, improves mental health, and likely increases lifespan. One of my favorite sentences comes from a meta-study in the *Journal of the American College of Cardiology*. "Running, even 5 to 10 minutes a day, and at slow speeds, is associated with markedly reduced risks of death from all causes and cardiovascular disease." If you're able to run but you haven't run today, find some time just to go around the block.

Many people believe there is some Goldilocks amount of exercise: not too little and not too much. Most things in life have limits. Driving 20 mph on a winding road will get you to your destination faster than driving 10 mph; going 100 mph will probably end badly. Friar Laurence's admonition to Romeo—"Therefore love moderately; long love doth so; Too swift arrives as tardy as too slow"—is one I've heard at many dinner tables and at least one TED Talk.

The data is mixed, but it generally favors the idea that running at any speed or distance is good for you. Yes, running long distances puts you at increased risk for atrial fibrillation, a rhythmic disturbance of the heart that increases your risk of a stroke. When you exercise frequently, your heart muscle grows larger. This growth can lead to stretching and damage. In a decade-long study of tens of thousands of skiers who participated in the arduous Vasaloppet cross-country skiing race in Sweden, the participants who had done it the most often and the fastest seemed to have the highest risk of atrial fibrillation.

But another study of a larger set of Vasaloppet skiers had another interesting finding: the more times people completed the intense ski race, the longer they lived. And the faster they completed it, the longer they lived. Michael Joyner, a distinguished sports physiologist at the Mayo Clinic, told me in an interview that there just doesn't appear to be any point at which increasing exercise increases overall risk of mortality. Yes, some risks go up. But so many other risks go down that you're still likely to live longer. Exercising some is clearly good, and exercising a lot is probably better. Don't just run around the block once; do it as many times as you can.

Running does all kinds of good things for your body: it keeps your weight down and it gets you outside. When I'm paying attention to my running, I eat more healthily than when I'm not. If I've gone for a run during the day, I'm more likely to fall asleep easily. My father's years of marathoning must have extended his life, somewhat. He stopped, though—perhaps because his body was just too broken down, or perhaps because he just didn't believe in himself any longer.

■

In 2016, my father sent an email while feeling particularly depressed. He wrote, "I'm in a corner. No Exit. I don't want to die begging. I've had 17 wonderful years more than Roger Hansen had when he came to this point. My body is 60, but my legs and hands are held together with wires and my head is full of Teflon. It's time to do the necessary."

This was a hard time in my father's life. He was 74 years old and worn down. His hands were cragged and bent from arthritis and years hunched over a keyboard. His liver was worn out from six decades of hard labor. He had lost most of his hair and dyed the last tufts an odd shade of rusty red. His teeth were rotting; his toenails were mostly black. He had had three hip operations and another surgery to fix a nerve issue near his brain. If he wanted to walk for any distance, he had to do it in a pool. One day, he found himself sitting in his car for 30 minutes struggling to breathe. He was living in Bali, and that night, at

3 A.M. his time, he sent me an email with the header "saying thanks in the twilight zone." He wanted to tell me how much he had loved spending time with me in my 20s, and to apologize for some of his behavior then. He couldn't wear happiness easily, he said, because he'd always had to fight so hard for his place in the sun. I read the email more in sorrow than in fear. He often talked about premonitions of the end. I was used to the drama. I responded quickly and kindly with a photograph of my three boys eating chips and guacamole.

In another gloomy email, he wrote that he was thinking back to me running with him in Boston: "Memories keep coming back, old age. Little boy joining me last half km of jog." I had just run a 2:46 in the New York City Marathon, and he sent me a short note saying "congrats on an excellent run" and then told me he was having trouble logging in to his account on newyorker.com. I offered my thanks and sent him his username and password, though I had given him a new one, "brandon," the name of our shared dog, to replace the most recent one he had used, "libido69."

Around this time, he wrote me that he needed a $1,500 bridge loan to cover hotel expenses in Malaysia. He'd been charged double for a flight he took and there was some confusing complexity involving a new boyfriend. He had some art he could sell, he claimed, and he promised to pay me back soon with interest. I knew he wouldn't, and I was frustrated. I told him, perhaps too coldly, that I didn't feel comfortable being a lender of last resort. I suspected that the problem wasn't the price of the hotel but rather the price of the man. He immediately wrote to my older sister, CCing me, and declared that he was cutting me out of his will and that suicide was at hand.

He had already taken the pills. His death, he wrote, "will give all of you a sigh of relief, one in particular." He sent another note to my older sister and me: "May you find as much happiness as I've enjoyed in recent years." I called him and then paid the hotel bill. Soon everything was fine, and he was sending cheerful emails again. The hotel, he noted, had a very cool book on guitars that he thought I should get.

It wasn't the only time he threatened to kill himself to wrangle a couple of hundred dollars out of me. Just as if he were a child, I knew that he loved me deeply and needed me, but I could only handle the manipulation in doses. Families are the only relationships that are permanent by definition. You can lose a best friend or leave a spouse. But your father will always be your father. This creates different obligations, frustrations, and kinds of love. It made me respond with empathy, but not in an unlimited amount.

The last email exchange I had with my father came in January 2017. I had just given him a birthday present of two books, and I had just gotten the job as the editor in chief of *Wired*, which my father mistakenly thought meant we were going to move west. He sent me an email with the subject line "everything." He thanked me for the books and for the bond we had developed over the decades. He was going to see a doctor and hoped, at the least, that his cardiologist would have good news. "I hope to send good news of sound body as in the past 5 (indeed the cardiologist usually bitches at his nurse for bringing X-rays of a 55 year old man). Marathons were a good investment."

He went on into deeper terrain, repeatedly referencing the biological roots of his sexuality, which he called his DNA-imposed limits, and his career frustrations.

Despite the separation in our family necessitated by something difficult with which to deal—in my DNA no less—we managed to develop some remarkable bonds.... You helped me through a most difficult period at midlife.... You went to Andover and Stanford—it's selfish but I hope Ellis does likewise.... You now rise far above what I even dreamed of, professionally (once I'd accepted my DNA imposed limits). We are all so proud. (But plz give *Wired* a New Yorker-style one page table of contents ... it is so tedious to peruse the magazine now).

You five will soon live in San Francisco the city of everyone's dream. I hope the condo trades nicely for the Paris-priced houses from which you select, as I assume you'll live in Pacifist Heights. Zachary will run up and down every almost-vertical street.

I know Danielle is giving up the most, but I know she will find the compensations. You are surely blessed by the gods in finding her (or as I understand, her finding you).

Reread the 23rd book of the Iliad, when the gods throw ashes on some and gold on others; destiny, and you got all gold.

I realize—painfully—that in a flat reversal of Asia, where money goes up, you grew up in a culture where it goes down; and I've had nothing for you and in fact the painful reverse.... my heart pounds with pride. Maybe my half of your DNA has been worth something along the way. It's enough for many lives.... I'm inherently happy and positive about life; ready to die fulfilled, hoping with good reason to have 15 more. Proudly, happily, Love Dad.

I sat in the purple chair in our apartment, reading the email over and over. I responded about an hour after I got the message, pleasantly but briefly. I tried to cheer him up by talking about the kids. I wanted them to get to know him. Two weeks later, at about 11 P.M., I got a note on Facebook Messenger telling me to call a foreign number. Part of me knew immediately what it meant. I rang and heard a male voice with a Filipino accent explaining that my father had died of a heart attack. The voice assured me there was nothing that could have been done. I said that I wasn't sure I had heard him correctly, even though I had definitely heard him correctly. Then I asked whether they were certain he was gone. The voice paused. Yes, they were, he responded, with a touch of incredulity, as though I had just asked if they were certain that rain had made the ground wet. My father would be buried in the Philippines as soon as my sisters and I could get over there. I walked to the bathroom, kneeled on the cold marble floor, and threw up into the toilet. Then I stumbled down the long, narrow hallway to tell Danielle. I called my sisters and then my mother. As in all moments of crisis and pain, she was as loving as could be.

Often the loss of a parent takes a long time. There are days spent in a hospital and then in hospice. A sudden death, however, makes everything quick and sharp. I had to make choices about the funeral. I had to tell my children that they had lost someone important whom they barely knew. I had to figure out the consequences of the half-baked will he had written, which gave away things he didn't have and provided no guidance on the things he did. I had to get on a plane to Manila. But really, I had to figure out how to process life now that one of the two people who had loved me every minute of it was gone. I had many other people I cared about, and many other people cared for me. But from this moment onward, I would always be more alone.

■

In the weeks and months after my father's death, I often found myself staring at a print by the twentieth-century American artist Ben Shahn. It had been my father's, but he'd given it to me in my 20s as partial payment for a loan. I had hung it on the wall above the philodendron that my mother gave me when I left for high school. The print renders, in Shahn's exquisite block calligraphy, a passage from Maximus of Tyre's *The Dissertations,* likely written in the second century AD, that my father has called his life's philosophy. Above the text, Shahn has drawn six simple faces, all in profile, gazing off to the side, as if searching for something just out of view.

> God Himself, the father and fashioner of all that is, older than the Sun or the Sky, greater than time and eternity and all the flow of being, is unnamable by any lawgiver, unutterable by any voice, not to be seen by any eye. But we, being unable to apprehend His essence, use the help of sounds and names and pictures, of beaten gold and ivory and silver, of plants and rivers, mountain-peaks and torrents, yearning for the knowledge of Him, and in our weakness naming all that is beautiful in this world after His nature—just as happens to earthly lovers. To them the most beautiful sight will be the actual lineaments of the beloved, but for remembrance sake they will be happy in the sight of a lyre, a little spear, a chair, perhaps, or a running ground, or anything in the world that wakens the memory of the be-

loved. Why should I further examine and pass judgment about images? Let men know what is divine. Let them know: that is all. If a Greek is stirred to the remembrance of God by the art of Phidias, an Egyptian by paying worship to animals, another man by a river, another by fire—I have no anger for their divergences; only let them know, let them love, let them remember.

I loved the print because of its beauty and because of the way it helped me understand my father's openness to experience. He moved between worlds with ease. The son of a Baptist minister, he claimed to be mostly Buddhist even as his world in his final years consisted mainly of Filipino Catholics and Balinese Hindus. He found wonder in music (the sight of a lyre) and in architecture (a chair). Danielle and I had had a multifaith wedding. Her mother is Catholic and her father is Jewish. My mother is a devout Episcopalian. I emailed my father to ask how he wanted his religious views represented, and he replied simply, "My favorite religious statement is on the Ben Shahn you have."

It wasn't until after his death that I noticed the three words that seem the most significant: "*a running ground.*" Among all the objects that could evoke memory and love, Maximus of Tyre included an ancient Greek track. My father must have seen these words hundreds of times as he studied the passage. Did he notice them? Did he think about how running had been one of the ways he had sought transcendence? Did he recognize that he had passed this particular quest on to me?

I realized, while focusing on those words, that running has long been a way for me, as Maximus of Tyre writes, to waken the memory of the beloved. When I run, I feel things more intensely. When I feel things intensely, I often feel like I'm running. As soon as I really focused on these three words, there was only one thing I wanted to do. I headed into the Catskill Mountains and ran for hours through the Burroughs Range.

Let them know. Let them love. Let them remember.

CHAPTER 11

Beet Juice

ME: How many hours a week do you think I train?
JAMES, AGE EIGHT: Thirty-five.
ME: Do you think I should train harder or less hard?
JAMES: Do you train mostly when I'm home or not?
ME: It's both. But a lot is when you're at school or when you're asleep.
JAMES: You should train harder when I'm not home, and not at all when I am.

A LITTLE MORE THAN A YEAR AFTER THE DEATH OF MY FATHER, I GOT AN email from an executive at Nike. The company was creating a new program that would pair regular runners with elite coaches, and they were wondering if I might be interested in participating. I got the email midweek, but I didn't respond immediately. As a journalist, I'm intrinsically skeptical of the motivations of large companies, and it did not escape me that the editor of a technology magazine might not have been randomly selected for a program designed to promote technology. I also worried about putting too much time into the sport. When you have an exhausting job, is it really a good idea to commit more fully to your exhausting hobby?

That weekend, I headed north to Andover. It was my 25th

reunion, and I wanted to see old friends. I also wanted an excuse to go for a very particular run. I found a parking spot behind the gym and changed into my running clothes in the back seat. I headed down to the school's blue track, across the grass fields, onto Salem Street, and then onto the road that leads to a simple, alliterative piece of heaven called Holt Hill, where my teammates and I used to train. It's a rolling hill with a pine-needle path to the top, where you can see all the way to Boston.

Loss is one of the forces that structures life. When we are young, we lose pets and grandparents. Our favorite spot in the woods gets turned into condos. Tragedy strikes, and we lose friends and homes. As we age, the losses become more frequent and defining. For reasons that can only be random, my high school cross-country team had been a source of constant slow pain. Four members of that team died young, including Tim Roberts, one of my closest friends in high school. I ran the route we had run together, thinking about loss and about my father.

I decided that I wanted to try to be fast again. I didn't have the words for it then, but running that route helped me realize that running faster would help me process my father's death. When you lose someone close, you can hold on through photographs. You can share stories, and you can cry. But sometimes you need to feel the person's presence, which isn't easy when the person's gone. Maybe you play chess, if that's what you did together. Or maybe you sit quietly in the chair where someone used to read to you. Or maybe you go and run. I couldn't go back and circle the boxwoods again. The dirt roads I had run with my father in Virginia had long since been paved. The house at the farm had collapsed. I could, though, insert a new intensity into a sport that I would forever associate with him.

So, I wrote to Nike and said that I was in. I would do the experiment. I would put in time and effort like never before. My father, of course, had wanted me to try to be better and more ambitious at everything, always. He would unquestionably have said to try this.

■

A few weeks later, I got on a conference call with Nike's three experts—Stephen Finley, a bighearted coach with the height of a basketball player and the patience of a watchmaker; Joe Holder, a physical trainer with the physique of a Michelangelo and the diet of a tortoise whose clients included Naomi Campbell and Virgil Abloh; and Brett Kirby, a sports scientist with the calm demeanor and seeming wisdom of Obi-Wan. I didn't know it then, but Kirby had designed some of the training for Eliud Kipchoge and can be seen on a bicycle in a YouTube video of one of the great Kenyan's marathons. People with credentials are often boring or cold. But each of these three men combined kindness with their wisdom. I would have happily left my kids with any of them for a day of homeschooling.

I told them how I'd trained in the past and what my goals were for the future. I explained that my marathon times had been remarkably consistent for more than a decade. I had finished both my first two NYC Marathons in 2:43 before Ellis was born. After Zachary, and then James, arrived, I had finished them in 2:42, 2:42, 2:45, 2:46, 2:46, and 2:43. One of my friends gave me a nickname: "Mr. Two Four Three." I hated it, but it was fair.

I told them that I loved the sport, and I wanted to understand it better. I would happily train smarter, I added, but I didn't have the time to train more. I sent them a link to my old online logs and told them that I now tracked every run on Strava. I told them that aging made me feel like a tire slowly deflating in the cold. They assured me that with science and a little bit of math, there was a way to pump some air in. They would work up a training program and put it all in a Google Doc. I told them that I wanted to break the idiosyncratic goal of 2:43 because it was two hours, plus my age in minutes. "My dream would be to run under 2:40," I said with a chuckle, "but there's no way I could go that fast."

That didn't have to be true, Kirby reassured me. As a person ages, he explained, the variables that control how fast we run don't ineluctably get worse. We often gain weight, but we can lose it again. We pick up bad habits from injuries that change our form—say, a tweaked right ankle that makes us land too hard on our left. But a habit caused by an unconscious choice can usually be reversed by a conscious one. Crucially, as Kirby explained, our muscles change in ways that are both good and bad. Our lean muscle mass declines with age, which is bad for marathoners and even worse for sprinters. We lose what is called peak propulsive force, meaning the power with which we push our feet into the ground. Our maximum heart rate declines. But as we train, over time, the mitochondria inside our muscle cells become more efficient at converting energy. New blood vessels develop. Tendons strengthen. We should, perhaps, get wiser.

Runners tend to decline badly in their 30s and 40s, but the main reason we slow isn't our bodies. It's our lives. We get married, we have children, we work longer hours, our parents get sick. We have more pressing things to do with our time. Running is a sport that rewards consistent effort, and once you step away, it's hard to come back. Your body frays, which makes running less enjoyable, which accelerates the decline. People stop running because they get old; they also get old because they stop running.

My new coaches listened to my description of the training regimen I had followed through my 30s and told me what it lacked. The long runs I was doing were good. The total volume of training—about fifty miles a week—was OK. Ideally, I'd run more, but changing that variable increases the risk of injury. There was one variable I could truly improve: time spent running *fast*. I wasn't doing remotely enough work to improve one of the key metrics of running: VO_2 max, a number that describes the body's ability to move oxygen through the blood during intense exercise. Or to put it in a formula: maximum milliliters of oxygen consumed in one minute divided by bodyweight in kilograms. Nor was I doing enough to improve my lactate threshold, a measure of the body's ability to move without the amount of lactate increasing in the blood. If VO_2 max is equivalent to a car's engine size, a runner's lactate threshold is the red line on the tachometer. I needed to improve both.

VO_2 max improves mostly through speed workouts—running quarter-miles, or miles, to the point of near exhaustion, resting briefly, and then running them again. Lactate threshold improves most through what are called threshold runs: running at a pace that's tiring but where you can still talk, at least a little. So, starting in early July, I began a new routine. I still got most of my miles in by commuting to and from the office, which was four miles away, on foot. But on Tuesdays I added focused runs to tax my VO_2 max, and on Thursdays or Fridays I added threshold runs. I started doing core workouts that Holder prescribed for me. A couple of times, I met him in gyms in Manhattan and he'd teach me how to properly do exercises I'd long neglected, from airplanes to pull-ups to Z-presses. He was astonished to learn how little I knew and to discover that I had the flexibility of the Tin Man.

Finley became the person I spoke with most. He wrote out plans for every workout in a Google Doc grid, and I would report each day how I'd done. He'd check it every now and then, and we'd talk every two weeks. Within a month, something had started to change. I was running mile repeats faster than I had done since college.

I wasn't following the prescribed program precisely, because life always intervened. I often had to run with a fanny pack to transport my wallet and keys, or a backpack to carry my clothes, which slowed me down. Sometimes I'd have to join a conference call while running, which slowed me down more. One afternoon when Danielle was working, I took my three sons to supervise my track workout, which was short-circuited when James, then four years old, justifiably declared himself bored and the workout over. Other runs involved stops at the dentist, the dry cleaner, and soccer practice. Red-eyes scuttled planned runs, as did sudden HR crises. But the Google Doc that Finley had made was forgiving. I just had to hit a few workouts precisely every seven days, and I had to get the weekly mileage roughly right. The rest was flexible enough for a man with a job, who had a wife with a job and three children with whom spending time was always an absolute joy.

The second big change in my routine came from data. I'd long believed that any data beyond the basic was a distraction. The quantified self is often a neurotic soul. For years I kept track of my runs with my stopwatch and guesstimated the number of miles I ran. Kirby persuaded me to break this habit.

Soon I was running with a Garmin Forerunner 935 on my wrist, an external heart-rate monitor attached to my arm, and little pods attached to both my shoes and my waistband that measured my power output and balance. After a run, I'd sync the Garmin and study the data. I now had precise information on how much of my energy had been spent going forward and how much I'd wasted swaying side to side. I could see how my feet had pronated and whether my heart had been beating as fast as it had during a similar workout two weeks before.

Kirby's training philosophy matched in many ways my favorite philosophy of playing music, often ascribed to Charlie Parker: learn all the theory you can, but forget it when you play. He wanted me to gather data. And he talked to me about "bottlenecks." Every runner has unique limitations: some physiological, some psychological, some biomechanical. The key isn't to try to improve everything at once, but to identify the current constraint and work to remove it. "You remove one bottleneck," he told me, "and then there's another. You only do what's necessary, so you widen your bottle to the next one." But as you do all that, he said, you have to stay in touch with why you love the sport. He was like a math wizard who also studied Zen philosophy. "I want the athlete to feel it," he said. "I don't want them to chase a metric on some device."

In mid-August, I traveled to Portland, Oregon, where I met Kirby in person. I walked on a mat that measures pressure and impact and learned that I land heavily on my forefoot, transition heavily to my heel, and then off again from my forefoot. The middle of my foot, it seems, does nothing. I did a test of ankle flexibility. I strapped on an oxygen mask, which made me look and feel a bit like a chemical inspector. Then I was put on a treadmill, facing a wall of white molds of the feet of famous athletes. I ran at increasingly faster speeds—starting at seven minutes per mile and progressing to 5:10 per mile. I would stop every three minutes so that Kirby could pluck a little blood from my fingers and measure how much lactate had accumulated.

Holder, meanwhile, instructed me on my diet. I'd always been reasonably healthy: staying away from junk and rarely ordering dessert. Holder said I needed, however, to change my frame of reference. I shouldn't just be avoiding bad foods. I should be actively seeking out good ones. I started to log every meal and every snack, a process that increases discipline in and of itself. I created a special breakfast that I ate every day, filling a huge glass container with seven days' worth of oatmeal, nuts, chia seeds, flaxseed, wheat germ, and bits of dried fruit. I shook it up every morning and poured a bowl that I topped with fresh fruit and milk. I usually followed that with a glass of green juice to help my gut and my immune system. I took L-citrulline pills, which Holder said would help with recovery. I tossed kale salads with protein and as many different colored vegetables as I could at lunch. At dinner, I joined in whatever we were eating as a family and tried to steer it in as healthy a way as I could. If we ordered burritos, I'd get a vegetarian one in a whole wheat tortilla without cheese or sour cream. I'd try to limit myself to one beer or glass of wine in the evening and then reach for kombucha if I wanted a second. The body builds and repairs muscle while we sleep, so I started to drink protein shakes before bed. I bought a two-liter water bottle and tried to finish it before I left work each evening. Holder also instructed me to drink beet juice every day. Beets contain nitrates, which your body converts into nitric oxide. Nitric oxide seems to increase blood flow and stamina. I ordered a case, stashed the little bottles in the fridge, and started popping one every morning. They tasted like sludge, and it was unnerving to pee red, but that seemed well worth it if I could get just a tiny bit faster.

I would later come to realize that all these interventions that the coaches were prescribing weren't just about my body, they were also very much about my mind. The point isn't merely to put more nitrates into the system. It's to remind someone that simple things exist that could make them faster. If you've found one, maybe it's time to seek out another: if you give a mouse a bottle of beet juice, he might just ask for a foam roller to use afterward. If he uses a foam roller, he might just start to think he can go quite a bit faster than 2:43.

■

The marathon, like so much else in life, is an event of small, imperceptible traumas that accumulate. I feel almost no fatigue between miles 5 and 10. But as I run forward—through Brooklyn, through Framingham, at the left corner of Lake Shore Drive, past the Cutty Sark—small muscle tears are accumulating in my legs. My body temperature is rising. I start to sweat in order to cool, but sweating only helps if the sweat can evaporate, which is hard when the air around me is humid. I start to breathe more quickly, decreasing CO_2 levels in my blood and slightly constricting the blood vessels that go to the brain. If I'm going even a tiny bit faster than the level known as my lactate threshold, my body is releasing hydrogen ions into the blood, making it more acidic. Lactate builds up, which isn't a problem in and of itself. But it's a sign of the baleful processes going on inside. Nerves in my legs are sending information up my body about damage and pressure. My store of carbohydrates is slowly depleting. No matter how much water I drink, I'm gradually becoming dehydrated. As I become dehydrated, it becomes harder for my body to transport oxygen through my blood to my muscles.

As I go, my brain is measuring all this and running a series of complex calculations just out of reach of my conscious mind. We often think of pain as something that happens in our bodies and then travels to our minds. That's true if you slide off a slippery rock and your ankle snaps. But I don't think the pain in running usually works this way. Instead, as a number of scientists have recently shown—and as two of my favorite authors, Alex Hutchinson and Steve Magness, have written—pain is also a psychological phenomenon. We feel it because the brain is telling the body to stop or slow because it's worried. The sports physiologist and ultrarunner Tim Noakes has called this phenomenon "the Central Governor Model." The title of his highly influential paper laying out this theory begins: "Fatigue is a brain-derived emotion."

One of the studies that most clearly shows this was conducted on a group of trained cyclists who were monitored in a laboratory under hot and cool conditions. From the beginning, the cyclists in the heat reduced their effort, even before there was any physical indication of fatigue and even before their body temperatures had started to rise. Their unconscious minds were apparently telling their bodies to take it easy for fear of what was to come. Noakes has said that his best evidence is the fact that so many runners are able to sprint at the end of a long race, particularly if they realize they are close to a goal. Their brains have told them that they're completely out of gas, until they realize the end is actually quite near, at which point the brain seems to let the body tap into a reserve. Another study showed that runners who swish a sports drink in their mouths—even if they don't swallow it—perform better. The brain seems to sense that nutrition is available, which temporarily reduces concerns about fatigue.

It seems that, while we run, our brains are making a series of calculations: measuring temperature, buildup of hydrogen ions, oxygen levels, electrolyte concentrations, muscle damage, our fuel stores, and more. Meanwhile, we're tracking our splits and measuring how we feel compared to how we expected to feel. We're subconsciously analyzing how far we have to go and how much damage to our bodies we've already done. I sometimes think of the brain as a thermostat, measuring hundreds of factors and combining them into some kind of "should we make Nick hurt" score. When the score gets too high, the thermostat sends a signal to fire up the pain furnace. That's when I ache and start to slow.

The goal of training isn't to try to unplug the thermostat, which is there for a reason. In a creative, if slightly psychotic, 2008 study, researchers gave cyclists fentanyl to block feedback during a time trial on exercise bikes. The riders had no understanding of their level of exertion so they rode at blistering speeds, faded precipitously, and couldn't walk afterward. That's what happens when the thermostat is off. Instead, my goal in training is to strengthen and stress all the systems that the thermostat is measuring to the same degree that those systems will be stressed on race days. I run down mountains, which tears my quads the way they'll tear on race day. I do 20-mile runs without drinking water or eating breakfast so that my glycogen stores and hydration levels will reach the levels of depletion I'll hit when I have prepared properly and run 26.2. I run when it's hot, when it's cold, when it's humid, when it's dark, when I'm hungry, and when I'm full. I run loads of miles at 5:30 pace even when I'm planning to run the race at 5:50 pace. I do this all for physical reasons: I want my body to be stronger, so it sends fewer signals to the thermostat. But I'm also doing it for psychological reasons. I don't want depletion of any of these systems to scare my brain. I want the bottlenecks to be wider and the thermostat set higher.

The Central Governor Model theory of fatigue also leads to an interesting hypothesis. Maybe one way to train ourselves to run fast is to train ourselves to endure in other tasks. As Hutchinson writes, endurance is what you need to finish a marathon and it's also what you need to fly cross-country with toddlers. To the extent that this is true, it gives me a theory for how to merge my hobby with my life. Long conference calls and stressful debates about the org chart are ways of learning to stay focused deep into a marathon. And staying focused deep into a marathon is a helpful way to learn how to stay calm and engaged two hours into a tense all-hands session.

The logic of the Central Governor Model also suggests that it can be helpful to trick yourself. That was the secret of that day on the Moses Brown track, when I broke through as a high school runner. I wasn't familiar with the track, and my brain didn't know it had to slow me down. The Central Governor Model suggests a mind-body dilemma. We all can go faster. We just need to persuade our brains not to start the subconscious shutdown process right away. But the only thing we can use to trick our brains is our brains. Training becomes a game of hide-and-seek with oneself.

■

When I started running in high school, I didn't care much about shoes. My coach soon directed me to buy my first pair of racing flats. These were soft and light: an extension of my legs, not a support for them. For the first time I could really feel my feet while I was running. My toes kissed the track and then propelled me forward. Outdoors, I screwed little spikes into the soles that conferred upon me control and power. Wearing those new shoes, my calves achieved more definition. I wasn't exactly a campus sex symbol: once, at Milton Academy, the fans in the stand started chanting "That boy has no butt! That boy has no butt!" as I raced to victory around the oval. Still, I felt a new physical confidence that ran from my feet upward.

After I left the track team at Stanford, I didn't buy another pair of racing flats for over a decade. I wanted cushioning for running long miles on the roads, convinced that my various aches and pains could be prevented if I strapped to my feet the closest thing I could find to a pillow. Once I joined the Central Park Track Club, though, my teammates educated me in the science of footwear. When a runner lifts their leg after it hits the ground, the motion resembles that of a pendulum, meaning that the mass of a shoe matters more than mass anywhere else on the body. An extra pound in your midsection will be less of a hindrance than 50 extra grams on your shoe. So, I started racing again in flats, even in the New York City Marathon, running across the Verrazzano in slipper-like shoes. The ideal shoes, the joke went, would disintegrate over the course of the race until they entirely disappeared as you crossed the line. These made you fast, but it cost you the ability to walk down the subway steps for several days after the race.

I began studying the ways that different shoes support different kinds of bodies, which seems obvious, but also the ways in which they interact with different surfaces, which isn't. Running on something hard, like concrete, loosens our bodies as we spring forward. Running on something bouncy, like wooden boards or a soft track, makes our bodies stiffen. Shoes are portable surfaces that you attach to your feet. But then, it's as hard to run with thick shoes on sand as it is to run barefoot on concrete. For each runner, with each distinct form, on each kind of terrain, there is an ideal shoe.

In 2017, Nike introduced the biggest breakthrough in distance footwear in a generation. It was called the Zoom Vaporfly 4%, and it had been secretly worn by three of the six men and women who qualified for the U.S. Olympic marathon team the previous year. These shoes used a new kind of foam, called PEBAX, generally found in airplane insulation. This made them well cushioned but also fantastically light. The Vaporflys weighed 190 grams each, about half as much as my regular training shoes. Inside each sole was a carbon-fiber plate that looks something like a spoon. The plate bends on impact, storing a bit of energy that it then offers back as propulsive force. It may even help stabilize the ankles. Critics called it illegal, which just made demand for the shoes go up. I got an early pair and was immediately convinced. They were hard to walk in, but they felt glorious to run in. I could go faster, and my legs hurt less afterward. Within a few years, every other major shoe company was copying the design and catching up.

Because I was part of the special program, I ran in these shoes, as well as in the special lightweight AeroSwift singlet designed for Eliud Kipchoge, then the world-record holder in the marathon. A shirt seems simple, but it needs to perform a variety of functions. It has to help the body cool itself by letting it sweat and then letting the sweat evaporate. It needs to minimize the torso's wind resistance. It needs to be light, and it really must not stick to your skin. One of Kipchoge's singlets had little spikes around it that, in wind tunnel tests, reduced the impact of wind. Mine had a big opening in the back to help with cooling. Relatively few people had worn this particular singlet, and it gave me a perverse thrill to know that I would be running the slowest marathon the shirt had ever seen.

I trained with Nike's coaches through August and September until, finally, in early October, I was ready to race the Chicago Marathon. The pace I could run in workouts was faster than it had ever been. I felt strong and my body had changed. Part of my job at *Wired* included appearing about once a week on *CBS This Morning* to talk about technology. I started to get emails from friends who had seen me, asking if I was OK: I was looking a little too skinny. I would smile and just write back that I had a race coming up.

The day before the marathon, I met my coaches in a cramped hotel conference room in downtown Chicago. Kirby pulled out a chart showing my overall fitness and level of fatigue, both derived from my Garmin data. It included details as precise as my speed going around turns. He showed me that my fitness level had been climbing since early July, and it had leveled off in the past 10 days while I had started to ease off my training in a blissful taper. But my fatigue was starting to decline, and performance, Kirby posited, depends on fitness minus fatigue. That number was at its peak.

Next, Kirby plugged my training data into a map of Chicago overlaid with the weather. It seemed to him and Finley that I should finish perhaps a bit under 2:39. Sometimes, the value of external validation is that it allows for internal validation. I could feel that the training had gone well. But without the data, and the experts examining the data, I would have been full of doubts about how I could do. I often sleep poorly the night before a race; that night, I drifted off with ease.

The morning was cold and windy, the start crowded as always, and I began much too slowly. I'm generally cautious early in a marathon, and I went through the first mile in 6:35, a pace that would put me across the finish line in 2:52. By mile 4, I had picked it up and was clicking off miles at between 5:57 and 6:04. I ate gels when I needed to; I tucked in behind groups when I could. My children cheered me on at mile 9.

I went through the half in 1:19:30 and held steady until mile 20, where I started to slow. But Kirby was there by the side of the course and said I was doing just fine. Encouraged, I began to accelerate, and I crossed the finish line at 2:38:23, my fastest finish ever. I was as elated and astonished as I had been 25 years before when I had finally made it up to the top of Kinsman Mountain. Kirby took a sonogram of my thigh for a study on post-race muscle inflammation as I high-fived him and my other coaches. I took the train to meet my kids, and then we zipped off to the airport.

■

After the Chicago race, I rested for a few days. When I started running again, I felt surprisingly good. Since I had already paid to register for the 2018 New York City Marathon, I figured I might try to run it. Danielle and James hadn't made it to Chicago. I didn't think I'd ever be that fast again, and I wanted them to see me.

And so, for the 11th time in my life, I took the ferry out to Staten Island for the start. I didn't have many goals for this race besides getting to see my children where Union Street hits Atlantic Avenue. The boys were now ten, eight, and four. As I approached them, I scrolled back through different memories of this spot. First, Danielle alone on the side. Then she's there pregnant, but not visibly so; then with one child in a stroller; one kid in a stroller and one standing; then two standing children and one in a stroller; then, finally, she's there with three, all standing and cheering right where they should be. One of them is almost as tall as she is. I can see their signs. I can hear their screaming.

Parenting is suffused with regrets, confusion, and mistakes. But when I run by, I know my children are rooting for me to succeed with infinite love and enthusiasm. I don't know what they'll think of marathoners when they've moved out or when I'm gone. I hope, though, that one day in the future, in whatever cities they live, they stand on the sidelines of a major race, watching the runners flow by, remembering cold November mornings from a generation ago when their father, then strong and quick, ran by on Atlantic Avenue. I hope, too, that maybe they have absorbed some of the things that I've learned as I've trained. They don't really have a sense of the way I do my job: it's too confusing and too distant. Physical work makes much more sense. They can see how tired I am after a workout, and they can appreciate what it means to have run 20 miles before breakfast. Perhaps, I hope, there are subtle lessons about resilience, dedication, and commitment that I'm passing along.

I moved out to the sideline and high-fived Ellis, Zachary, and James's little palms, and blew a kiss to Danielle. Ellis, the oldest, handed me a little water bottle, and Zachary and James each gave me an extra gel pack, just as we had practiced while I ran around the dining room table in our apartment. I looked back briefly, and they were yelling me on. I ended up running another 2:38, which made it my fastest New York City Marathon. I rested for two months, and then I wrote to Finley and told him that I wanted to get faster still. He wasn't surprised. Runners never stop after setting a personal best. Finley wrote back and said of course he'd help.

My training rests on a series of routines: When I'm home in New York, I wake up at the same time, eat the same breakfast, and run four miles to the office. At the end of the day, I run home. Finley said to keep doing all this and just to train with a little more intensity, in every way. He created another plan in a Google Doc, and I began to follow the routine in earnest as the winter in New York started to bear down. Before Chicago, I had run an average of 55 to 60 miles per week, roughly half of what a professional marathoner does. By February 2019, I was up to 65 to 70 miles. On Tuesdays, I would do speed workouts, repeating circuits that were short and fast, like eight repeats of 1000 meters hard, with rests in between. Sometimes, Finley would have me run 20 repeats of shorter intervals, both to increase my speed and to get me mentally ready for a race that is broken up into 26.2 parts. On Thursdays, I would do tempo runs, meaning, for example, that I would do three repeats of a 2-mile circuit, with rests in between. On Sundays, I would run long. The schedule would usually call for between 16 and 20 miles, but I'd run a bit more. All the other days, he marked "run option," meaning I would do whatever I wanted. As I increased the intensity of the training, I also dropped things. When my mileage increased past a certain level, I stopped keeping track of my push-up and core workouts. Early in the cycle I ran barefoot from time to time to strengthen my feet. Late in the cycle, I wouldn't bother. In my job, I like to think about things called "non-goals": projects that are undeniably valuable but which I'm not going to do because I don't have the time. Anything I add to a to-do list has to be more important than the most important non-goal. The same principle applied to my new training. Sometimes, subtraction matters as much as addition.

I stayed as much on schedule as was possible, given the demands of my job. I was managing my team as the editor while also working on a series of stories with a colleague about Facebook that would become some of the most influential articles I ever wrote. This led to the occasional training hiccup. Traveling for work in Abu Dhabi, and stymied by sand and wind, I couldn't even run a six-minute mile. When I got back, I tried to do a long run in Prospect Park at night, and somewhere on the far side of the park, I pulled over by a water fountain and almost fell asleep on the ground not far from a raccoon. Another day, I took my racing shoes to the local track at the start of a snowstorm. Slick marathon shoes with carbon plates are good for many things, but these had the traction of a spoon wrapped in a banana peel. My marks in the snow were roughly left foot, right foot, left foot, butt print, arm print, left foot, right foot, butt print.

These hitches notwithstanding, I began to notice things getting better early on. During the previous training cycle, I'd fallen apart every time I ran a mile anywhere under 5 minutes and 35 seconds. Then, one day, I was racing down the drive in Prospect Park, drafting behind a guy riding a cargo bike. "Dude, how fast you going?" he asked. I looked down and was startled to tell him I was running at 5:25 per mile. He gave me a thumbs-up and kept on helping me out.

The real test came in April, at the Boston Marathon. I set my goals cautiously. Just maybe, I could break 2:35. But a canny marathoner has a private goal and a public goal. I told everyone I was trying to break 2:37:12, a marathon run at exactly a six-minute pace, which my high school cross-country coach had once told me was the cutoff time for a real runner. I went up the day before the race and stayed with my mother. I slept in a small room just off her library, a splendid and cavernous room lined wall to wall, and floor to ceiling, with art history books. The books were arranged by historical period, with sliding ladders so she could climb up and reach the ones on the top.

My mother wasn't particularly concerned with my various time goals. They were just numbers. She cared whether I was happy and that I had what I needed. She filled the fridge with beet juice before I arrived, because she knew I liked to drink it, but she had no idea how to answer when a friend of hers asked her how fast I was likely to run. She thought it might have been under three hours, but she wasn't sure. One of her greatest virtues has been her ability to maintain steadfast and absolute love for me along with total indifference to my win-loss record. She must have driven me to 200 soccer games and tennis tournaments when I was a child. She always got me there on time with my gear properly packed. But I don't remember her being concerned, a single time, with the score. She had come to watch me run the Boston Marathon once before and expressed surprise that I had just zipped by and waved. "I thought you were going to stop and chat," she said afterward. This time, I gave her a hug goodnight and told her precisely what time I would be passing by Boston College, where she planned to watch.

The gun went off, and everything flowed just fine. I ticked off the early miles exactly on target, and the hills passed much sooner than I expected. At one point, I went by one of my training partners who had started faster than I, gotten frustrated, left the course, and chugged a beer on the sideline. At 21 miles, just after Heartbreak Hill, my mother hollered words of encouragement. Soon I was racing downhill toward Kenmore Square. I ran mile 22 in 5:27 and finished the race at a new personal record of 2:34. I was now inhabiting a racing body that was entirely new.

■

My coach, Steve Finley, moved around a lot as a kid. His mother was a corporate executive at Kraft Foods and the family breadwinner. Every two years or so, she'd be offered a new assignment in a new city. Finley was born in Allentown, Pennsylvania. Then came stops in Nashville, Clarksville, Memphis, Ridgewood, Fayetteville, Syracuse, Cleveland, and back to Allentown. His father was a track-and-field coach and a stay-at-home dad. He'd get a job at a local high school in their new town and teach the kids to jump, throw, and run. Steve learned to throw a broom like a javelin as a kid. When he took up running, he was remarkably good.

Finley was an elite runner in high school and then at the University of Virginia. He transferred to the University of Oregon, where he ran for a year and learned the business of coaching from my Stanford coach, Vin Lananna. He qualified for the Olympic Trials in the steeplechase and had a shot to make the team, but, shortly before the race, he ruptured an Achilles tendon. The injury took years to properly heal, and it put an end to his dream of running professionally. Eventually, he moved to New York, built a team called the Brooklyn Track Club, and became one of the most respected coaches in the city. Nike signed him up for special projects.

Finley had learned the art of coaching through close observation and attention. He'd watched his dad figure out how to make the best out of awkward teenagers, and then he'd watched Vin Lananna train Olympians. He understood the physiology of training, and the psychology too. Anyone can give a runner a workout. But training is not math. Finley knew that a coach has to understand a runner's mind too.

Years after my success, I sat down with Finley at the Hungry Ghost coffee shop off Flatbush Avenue in Brooklyn. I wanted to know what secret tricks he'd used on me. He said he'd realized the key thing first. "You were intrinsically motivated," he said. "You had already built training into your day, your life, your family, your job. You loved to run . . . we needed to mentally convince you that you could step into this much younger, much more athletic version of yourself again because usually it's forgotten. That was the retraining of your mind." He knew that I was in my mid-40s but that my body wasn't as broken-down and didn't have the wear and tear of people who'd hammered 10,000 miles in college or raced hard in their 20s.

Immediately after our first conversation during the summer of 2018, Finley began working on his plan for me. First, he had me run short intervals and sprints. The goal was to improve my efficiency and form—and to get me used to running at much faster paces. He learned that I would do his speed workouts precisely as he put them in the Google Doc, and that I would disobey his directions for long runs. So, he wrote down the short workouts exactly as he wanted me to do them and sandbagged the long ones. He had one argument with Joe Holder, who thought I needed a much more aggressive active stretching and cross-training routine. Finley thought it might just screw me up after a lifetime of running one way. Finley won the argument, and, as a result, I still can't touch my toes.

Finley built a program that would work with my whole life, which is what the best kind of coach should do. "A big piece of my coaching philosophy is how can we accomplish that holistic experience from having a great family to doing great work? How does running add to all of this? And it should never stand in the way. My job is to make sure you can do all of this at a high level. It's not that you just have that one goal. It's all the goals." This was a profound insight, and it was, in retrospect, the only kind of coaching that would have worked for me. Running has never been the most important thing in my life. I've always cared more about family, about work, about many things. A coach who didn't see or couldn't accept that could never have gotten the best out of me. That's part of why I failed under Lananna and succeeded under Finley.

And the deal of course worked both ways. I run about 3,000 miles a year, and it takes about eight hours out of every week. There are days when my running annoys my wife, my children, or my colleagues. I've missed movies that Danielle has watched with the kids because I've gone off running; I've accidentally woken her up far too many times while heading out the door in the morning. I've annoyed my sisters by wearing myself out during morning workouts before family hikes. The list of minor infractions is long. One time, early in our relationship, I was at Danielle's parents' house. We had a family meal and then, at 10 p.m., I headed out for a run. After I had left, my future mother-in-law asked what on earth was wrong with me. "The thing you have to understand," Danielle said, "is that he enjoys it."

We basically have a deal. I try my best to make my obsession as minimally disruptive as possible. She rolls with the disruption and knows that I'll make it up to her in other ways. We have a marriage with balance, love, and trade-offs. Danielle and my children also understand both what running means to me and that I never let it become the thing that matters most. I might run while my kids warm up for their soccer games, and I might do planks during halftime. But when the game begins, I'm on the sideline cheering as loud as anyone else.

CHAPTER 12

2:29

ME: Does my obsession about running ever seem strange to you?
ELLIS, AGE 14: No. The green drink is nasty. But it doesn't bother me that you do planks when we watch movies.
ME: That's good.
ELLIS: After that Brooklyn marathon, where you had to curl up next to a space heater under a blanket on the floor, you seemed strangely content for someone who was clearly miserable.
ME: How long do you think I'll keep running?
ELLIS: As long as you can. Until your leg snaps for real.
ME: Do you think there's anything about it that has shaped you?
ELLIS: Probably. But I have no idea what.

THE SENSATION OF GROWING STRONGER IS ONE OF THE MOST BEAUTIful things about this sport. As my training intensified, everything about my body—and my awareness of it—sharpened. I would lie in bed at night, focusing on my pulse inside different muscles. I could trace the fatigue from my big toe to my hips. I particularly liked to focus on the broad ache in my hamstrings. They felt hot, filled with the last orange embers of a firepit. I came to find pleasure in the short, stiff steps I had to take whenever I stood up from my desk, and the slow, rickety shuffle with which I had to begin my runs. When your mitochondria are becoming more efficient, they need time to wake up. Finley had set my tachometer right on the red line: I was pushing as hard as I could without breaking. My body was tearing and growing, tearing and growing, but I wasn't getting hurt. Every day I felt stronger than I had the day before. My resting heart rate dropped and dropped. I eagerly checked each morning to see if it had fallen below 40 while I slept.

It didn't take me long to recover from the Boston Marathon that spring. Just one month later, I entered a half-marathon in Brooklyn and flew across Prospect Park and down Ocean Parkway at a 5:30 pace. I sprinted across the Coney Island Boardwalk and finished in 1:11, by far my fastest time at that distance. Sometimes success feels impossible; sometimes it feels inevitable. It was the seventh race I'd run since starting my training program with Finley and Nike a year before, and the seventh one in which I had exceeded my highest expectations.

I recovered briefly from the Brooklyn Half and then talked with Finley about a new goal: breaking 2 hours and 30 minutes at the Chicago Marathon in the coming fall. The idea would have seemed absurd to me a year before. My personal best had improved by four minutes in 12 years of relentless work. Now, with Finley's help, I was aiming to take it down by 10 minutes in 12 months, at an age where I was closer to social security than to college. Finley methodically planned workouts to slowly shift my physiology and my psychology too. He plotted everything out in a new Google Doc with workouts like: "6x 1 mile w/ 90 sec rest start at 5:50, 5:45, 5:40, 5:30, 5:25, 5:20." Every Tuesday, I would run long, hard repeats. Every Thursday, I would run short, even harder ones. On Fridays, I'd run a little bit longer and a little bit faster than usual. Every Sunday, I'd run long but not hard. I started doing short sprints after runs to increase the power of my stride. The point of the workouts was to tire me but not to obliterate me. There would be another workout in two days. As Ernest Shackleton famously remarked, it's better to be a live donkey than a dead lion.

As I progressed, I kept in mind one idiosyncratic goal: I wanted to win the Northeast Harbor Road Race. For every summer of my childhood, I had spent a month with my mother and sisters in this small town near Acadia National Park in Maine. There, every August, a five-mile race traverses one of the most beautiful routes in America. You start on Sargeant Drive and cover the first few miles on a narrow, curving road. On your right is Somes Sound, a fjord formed by glaciers that splits Mount Desert Island in half. It's an ocean with the spirit of a lake: deep and cold enough to be filled with lobsters, but small and bounded enough to be swimmable. On the left are the steep slopes of Little Brown Mountain. Rectangular boulders sit just to the cliff side of the road, stopping cars, bikes, and maybe runners from skidding off course and plummeting down to the lobster buoys. About two miles in, there's an eastern white pine, sculpted to perfection by man or by wind. It stands alone as perfectly balanced as a dancer raising her hands and lifting one leg gracefully back.

The course stays by the Sound for a third mile, but the water gradually fades from view. Soon you're running by the side of a golf course, across from mansions with tennis courts and lush hydrangeas. You pass the swim club and the sailing club. With less than a half mile to go, you turn left at the church, St. Mary's by the Sea, and begin to sprint to the finish line in the town's short main street, across from the Colonel's Restaurant. This is where I earned $3.65 an hour washing dishes the summer I turned 13. It still serves the best crullers I've ever had.

My father ran the Northeast Harbor Road Race once, in 1980. He finished in 33 minutes, a respectable time, but seven minutes behind the winner—Michael Westphal, a strapping young engineer from nearby Great Cranberry Island. I remember, when I was about 10, watching the runners as I stood by the swim club. A week or two later, I walked around my mother's vegetable garden vowing that I would win the race and plotting when that might happen. Maybe, I thought, in college. But victory proved elusive. I ran the race the summer before my freshman year at Stanford, at a moment of peak fitness, but came in third. In my late 20s and 30s, I ran it a few more times but my best finish was around fifth. In 2017, I came in third but befriended the winner, Judson Cake, a lanky policeman from nearby Bar Harbor. He was 39, three years younger than I, and it was his fourth victory. He had a mustache and a rhythmic running stride, with his upper body always moving gently right to left, left to right. We became training partners. He'd work all night, then meet me to train on the Acadia carriage trails at 8 A.M. We'd finish and he'd drive home to sleep through the day.

The summer after I'd trained with Finley and the others, there was no longer a gap between me and Judson. Two years before, I had stood on the starting line knowing I would lose. Anyone watching could have known it too. Judson had warmed up with confidence and stood right at the starting line with his head up; I had been fiddling with my watch, looking down, thinking already of the reasons why I wouldn't win. This year I looked and felt different. A race is never won at the starting line, but it can be easily lost. That wasn't going to happen here.

Judson and I took it out side by side, trading the lead every half mile or so. At about mile 3, I gradually pulled away. When I made the turn by St. Mary's, I heard footsteps and assumed that Judson had caught back up to me. But it was a young man wearing a Hawaiian shirt. Judson had faded back and would come in third. I was startled, but confident. I had wanted to win this race since well before my new competitor was born. I was able to sprint down Main Street and get away. My children, and nieces and nephews, were there screaming and dancing as I dashed toward the tape. It was only the second race I'd won in 26 years.

■

The next day, I ran with Judson through Acadia National Park. We traveled across a smooth gravel carriage road called Around Mountain, with the remnants of a giant glacial-era rockslide on the right and the shimmering waters of Jordan Pond down below. After about 16 miles, Judson decided to head back to his car. I turned and ran up and down Cadillac Mountain, giving me 25.6 miles for the day. Two days later, I ran 20 x 200 meters all-out on a track in Columbus, Georgia, where I was giving a speech about trends in technology. I was feeling great, and I had a month and a half to go before the Chicago Marathon.

The next six weeks were a period of precision and obsession. I monitored my weight, my heart rate, and my diet. I visualized each workout. I made sure to sleep eight hours a night. One day, Finley prescribed "5 mile progressive tempo starting at 5:50–5:30, 2 min rest, followed by 2 x 1 mile @ 5:20 with 2 min rest." I ran the five miles of the tempo run in 5:50, 5:44, 5:39, 5:32, and 5:26, and then I ran the two single miles in 5:16 and 5:09. One of the wonderful things about being in top shape is how in touch I feel with my body: I could run a mile on a flat road and, without looking at my watch, tell how fast I had run more or less to the second. I had expected to run the final mile of that workout in 5:10 and felt pleasantly surprised when my watch said 5:09. Finley wasn't just structuring the workouts to make me faster; he was also subtly training good racing habits. He always directed me to run the last mile faster than the first one. This is how you should run a marathon too.

The morning of the Chicago Marathon, I woke in my hotel and checked the weather report for the hundred and seventh time. Everything was perfect: it was cold and clear with little wind. I drowned myself in beet juice and, lacking utensils, used the knife on a hotel corkscrew to spread peanut butter on a bagel. I hydrated with water, dehydrated with coffee, and hydrated again. I watched my favorite race video: the great Kenyan Olympic champion Sammy Wanjiru outkicking his rival on the Chicago course nine years prior. Then I made my way to the start. Finley came, and he, Ellis, and my sister Heidi and her kids positioned themselves on the course at strategic spots to cheer me on. I spent some of the time before the race obsessing about the fact that I had brought two socks of slightly different sizes, but mostly I felt confident. If the day was perfect, 2:30 was possible. My sister Phyllis has always been in charge of my skin care, and she had given me a thick zinc oxide sunscreen, which I put on just before heading out the door. I didn't properly rub it in, which meant I had a slight zombie appearance as I left. None of the other runners—deep in their own worlds and micro-dramas—noticed. At least, none of them pointed it out.

The gun fired and I went off at a familiar speed. Finley wanted me to run the first half of the race at 5:45 pace, but the skyscrapers of Chicago intoxicated my GPS. I worried briefly, relaxed, and then passed the first mile marker at 5:45 on the nose. At times, as in all races, I felt exhausted and confused, and I wanted to puke or drop out. But mostly I simply tried to breathe, relax, and save energy by thinking about as little as possible. I latched on to the back of a group of elite female runners who I knew would keep a steady pace. Fans screamed "Let's go, girls!" at us.

I passed the half in 1:14:59. By mile 22, part of my brain was celebrating that I would likely break 2:30, and the other half was delineating all the things that could still go wrong. Then, at mile 25—pushing north on Michigan Avenue with Grant Park not far in the distance—I tried to accelerate and suddenly felt as if I were running in boots made of concrete. I felt momentary panic, the kind you get when your car first starts to skid on ice. But then I steadied myself and tried to concentrate on my breathing and the meditative pattern I sometimes use while running—counting out patterns of three as my feet hit the pavement. One, two, three. Right foot, left foot, right foot. One, two, three. Left, right, left. It's my version of a mantra, and the idea is to build one strong enough to cancel out the negative and untrustworthy thoughts of your tired mind. I thought about posture and trying to keep relaxed from the base of my skull to my heels, and from my cheekbones to my toes. I reminded myself that it didn't matter if I ended in a sprint, as long as I didn't end in a crawl. I visualized all the pain in my body and then imagined loading it into a wheelbarrow and pushing it away.

Hitting my goal meant running a marathon in 9,000 seconds, and I crossed the line with just 47 to spare: 2:29:13. There were some 46,000 finishers, only one of whom was both older and faster than I. My family sent texts full of emojis and love. Finley came running to congratulate me and celebrate, and he revealed that, having seen me the week before, and toward the end of the race, he'd worried I'd pushed it too far. For the first time, he said, I had looked like I was truly exhausted. But I'd made it. I'd done it. I told him I wanted to get right back at it. He suggested it was time to stop for a while.

Ellis had been able to come and watch the race. His younger brothers had soccer games. In the taxi to the airport afterward, I asked him what my next goal should be.

"2:35," he said.

"2:35?" I asked in surprise, thinking perhaps he had meant 10 minutes faster.

"You think you're going to run that fast again?" came the response, with wide eyes and a perfect grin.

■

After I ran 2:29, I tried to think deeply about why I had run so fast. Some reasons were obvious: I had run more miles, and I had run them hard. I wore carbon-plated shoes and drank beet juice. Some explanations were buried deeper. Steve Finley had wanted to unlock a younger version of me, and he had subtly done it. He had realized, just by talking to me on the phone in that first conversation, that I had more talent than I thought. But he couldn't tell me that directly. He had to guide me to that realization. Each of these things was important, but they didn't fully explain my speed. I wondered about the timing. My father had begun to run fast after his father died; I had started to run fast after my father died. In my case, that seemed more like a coincidence than a cause.

Then, one frosty morning a few months later, I was running my regular commuting route across the Brooklyn Bridge. I had walked James to school on Sixth Avenue and then turned to jog down through Brooklyn, winding through Park Slope, the

Gowanus Houses, and Brooklyn Heights. I cut through Cadman Plaza, running a few hundred meters on the lovely, rubberized path across from the Eastern District courthouse where, among other high-profile defendants, El Chapo had recently been tried. I passed a cluster of egg-sandwich and coffee stands and turned up the crowded steps to the Bridge. I was wearing my normal run-commute outfit: sweatshirt, Tracksmith running pants, and a red waist pack that held my cellphone, wallet, and keys. I had done this route around 2,000 times in my years of commuting to Manhattan. I was running slowly, as I almost always do on commutes.

At work, I usually shut down my senses. When I'm relaxing on a run like this, I try to open them. I try to sense the difference between the way my feet feel when I step on asphalt and concrete, or the brief, slightly scary, give I feel when I step on the metal grounding of a restaurant's loading entrance. I listen to the different sounds of cars, not just the buzz of the engines but the *pu-wow-clack* when a truck goes over a little bump. I feel the different rhythms of the day; some of my favorite city runs are in the early hours of sunrise as the fishermen head out and the young lovers head in. I smell the pretzel carts, taste the cold air in my mouth, and look at the remnants of a night well lived. New York City is unlike any other place in the world. The best way to experience it all is to crisscross it at dawn.

This morning, after drop-off, running down the bridge, with City Hall just ahead, a realization made me stop mid stride. My body, it seems, had figured out something profound before my mind could quite articulate it. I pulled off to the side and sat down on a metal bench, and then it came to me. I hadn't been able to run a fast marathon in the past *because I hadn't wanted to*. Or, more precisely, I hadn't really cared about going that fast because all I really wanted was something else. After my experience with thyroid cancer, all I had sought, deep down, was to be the person I was before I got sick. I had just wanted to match the Nick I had been before the diagnosis, training for the first time with the Central Park Track Club and running that glorious 2:43 before the doctor found the lump in my throat. Every year I could run that speed was another year that I knew I was still alive. This kept me going, but it also held me back. I had tried harder each year, but I only changed enough to keep everything the same.

As I glanced at Borough of Manhattan Community College and dodged a young tourist with a selfie stick, I thought about how long I had been satisfied to run 2:43 after 2:43 after 2:43. If I hadn't found Finley, I would never have figured that out. I looked out at the city and focused on a terrace on about the 50th floor in a giant apartment building across the street. On the terrace, a yellow kayak was resting in the cold sun. I had noticed it almost every day for years and thought of it with a certain amount of sadness—because the boat, as far as I could tell, had never touched water—and a certain amount of hope, because surely someday it would.

We all contain different versions of ourselves buried deep inside. This faster Nick had always been there, perhaps for 25 years. To find him, I had needed distance from the cancer, and I had needed Finley's plans. I wondered then, as I wonder now, what other versions of me exist that there may no longer be time to find.

■

The next Northeast Harbor Road Race came when Zachary was 11 years old and on a fiercely competitive soccer team. In June, we had started running on a track in the Catskills and he had done a mile in about 10 minutes. We went back every few days, and his time dropped and dropped. The kid inherited his mother's coordination and balance, along with my hair and trainability. My objective in parenting has always been to be there for the kids, but never to push them. I don't want to tell them to go run, or train more for soccer, or prep more for a debate tournament, but I always want to be there for them if they want it. Zachary clearly wanted to get faster, so I wanted to help him do it. I'd run in front of him and try to figure out from his breathing the fastest pace he could handle without getting frustrated. In mid-July, I drove him up to Boston, on our way to a sleep-away camp in Maine. The next morning, we stopped at a track nearby and I paced him to a 6:58 mile as my mother cheered him on.

After camp, he and I started running in Maine. We ran four miles together one day and then five two days later. It took us 56 minutes, and Zachary was exhausted at the end. "How much longer?" "A mile." Then, less than a minute later: "Are we almost there?" "No, there's still .9."

The morning of the Northeast Harbor race, he came into my bedroom and declared, "I am so ready for the race." I told him to eat a light breakfast and tried to get him to think about other things. We walked to the start from our house on Schoolhouse Ledge, and he laughed as I stepped gingerly onto the shortcut through the woods, trying not to scrape my racing shoes.

We registered and, as the winner of the last race, I was given bib #1 for the first time in my life. He was #49. I told him to warm up the way I warm up for a marathon: walk and stretch. But don't burn those energy stores. My friend Sarah Saint-Amand had promised to run with him at a pace of 10 minutes per mile. I set out on my regular warm-up. I ran two slow miles and then some strides as he stood and laughed with Sarah near the gas station. He didn't seem nervous at all.

We lined up and I reached back to give him a fist bump. Then: "On your marks. Go!" I did just fine and came in third, after Judson and a phenom from Williams College who was passing through town and dusted both of us. After finishing, I grabbed some water and ran the course in reverse, with Judson by my side. I looked for kids Zachary's age who he might want to pass. I saw none, though I did note a teenager in a Patagonia shirt, walking. I saw an older man weaving across the road, side to side. At first, I thought he was in trouble and perhaps having a stroke. But Judson said "he's fine," and I trusted his policeman's instinct. Right around mile 4, I saw the light-blue outline of a Manchester City jersey. It was Zachary, and he looked great. He was side by side with Sarah, smiling and looking strong. His form was good. I turned, pivoted, waved goodbye to Judson, and asked Zachary how he was doing. Good, he said. I ran with him and Sarah for a minute listening to his breath and his stride. He did seem OK, so I told him to push. Focus on the runners ahead of you and try to reel them in. Weirdly, I said "roll them in," but I didn't feel like correcting myself and assumed he got the point.

And then one by one he rolled them in. There was a woman in a hunter-green tank top off in the distance, and I told him to focus on her. We pulled closer and then Zachary told me his shoe was untied. We stopped, I double laced it, and off we went again. His breathing seemed good, so I told him to keep accelerating and catching people. By the last quarter-mile, he was in a near sprint and I turned off the course. His cousins started to scream and dance and wave the signs they had made for him: "Go Zachary. The God." He caught the teenager in the Patagonia shirt, who then started to sprint away. He finished in 44:53. Sarah followed right after. The man swaying from side to side came in directly behind them.

We celebrated with crullers at the Colonel's. He'd done something I hadn't been able to do as a kid. He was proud and flushed. I wondered whether this would be the moment that he would come to love the sport. Maybe, or maybe not. Either way, he had learned how to train and how to improve. The next day, Zachary declared that one day he was going to win the race. It was a vow, just like the one I had made walking in my mother's vegetable garden 35 years before.

Later that day, I texted Judson and asked if he knew the man weaving back and forth across the road near Zachary. "Yeah," Judson said. "He's Michael Westphal from Great Cranberry Island. One of the best runners from this state. He's got Parkinson's, but he's never stopped running." I looked in the race's historical results. Westphal had won in 1980, the year my father ran. Forty-one years later, Westphal had finished just behind my son.

CHAPTER 13

Michael Westphal

There's more to running than just beating people. I realized that when I was 58.

—MICHAEL WESTPHAL

A WEEK LATER, I TOOK A FERRY OUT TO GREAT CRANBERRY WITH ELLIS. Michael Westphal was at the top of the stairs of the dock to greet us. He was 64 years old, with a runner's thin build and thinning white hair. He wore a light turquoise shirt, white pants, and dark-blue New Balance shoes. He was shaking and swaying and jerking. He said hello and his voice seemed controlled, but his body did not. We got into his beige Subaru Outback, which he had driven as far as you could toward the dock. He leaned back, his head going side to side, his left arm swinging behind him and against the seat, and his legs jolting up to his chest. Up and down. Side to side. Up and down. It seemed impossible that he could drive, but he had gotten here. Surely, he could get back. I buckled my seat belt and we drove slowly off. Ellis would admit later that he too was terrified.

Great Cranberry Island is a sliver of beauty in a cold, tiny part of the world. It's two miles long and a mile wide. The year-round population is about 40. The island sits about 20 minutes by boat from the mainland. There's a single paved road that goes roughly north to south. Westphal grew up here, with three sisters and two brothers, in a house without heat. His father commuted to and from Boston, where he would stay three days a week, and his mother raised the family. Every few weeks, she would head off by boat and buy groceries. They stored a lot of powdered milk and kept the freezer full.

Westphal's best friend was the one other boy his age on the island, Gary Allen. They studied together in a tiny schoolhouse and roamed in the forest and on the rocky beaches. They learned improvisation, resilience, and all the other skills that someone bounded in a nutshell needs to become a king of infinite space. Allen, whose family could trace its roots on the island for 12 generations, back to the 1650s, took up running first. He watched Frank Shorter win Olympic gold in 1972 and decided he wanted to do that too. This naturally inspired Westphal, and it wasn't long before they realized they were both good. They trained together by running endless loops down and back on the main road. Two miles one way, two miles the other way. Over and over. The road starts at just about sea level and climbs to about 80 feet. Sometimes Westphal would take the side roads down and back. Allen liked to stay on the thoroughfare. Other islanders took to the sport as well. A tiny island can't field a soccer team.

Allen and Westphal led Mount Desert Island High School

to frequent victory and Westphal won the high school cross-country triple crown: individual glory, a team state championship, and getting the prettiest girl on the team, Jennifer, to date him. The next stop for Westphal was the University of Maine, where he ran a 4:19 mile. A few years after graduation, he married Jennifer, and they moved back to the island, where he started work as a carpenter. Allen, who had skipped college to start working as a lobsterman, was already there, running up to 150 miles a week, back and forth on the two-mile road. Westphal liked to keep it closer to 100. Small islands off the coast of Maine are not known for their hospitable winter weather, and I asked Westphal how many days the snow and ice kept him inside. "Never," he responded. "It's just a choice." He said that running on ice helped him develop a tremendous sense of balance.

The other islanders became obsessed with the sport too. Perhaps the success was osmotic: it's easier to be a fast runner when the only runners you know are fast. Perhaps it was cultural: training requires grit and perseverance, which are traits you learn quickly on an island, drinking powdered milk. Some of it was genetic: Westphal had two sisters and a brother who became excellent runners. Perhaps it was just because there wasn't that much else to do. You can't skip your run to watch a movie when there isn't a movie theater and you don't have a VCR. Whatever the reason, by the early 1980s, the island had six residents who were running sub-3-hour marathons. They all pushed one another. Allen would go out and look at Westphal's footprints in the snow and count how many laps of the main road he had run. From the spacing, he could tell how hard his friend had gone. Then Allen would try to go harder. Allen estimates that the island had the highest density of fast marathoners of any place in the world outside of Iten, Kenya.

Westphal and Allen started to take boats to the mainland and race wherever they could in Maine. Westphal was the faster of the pair, and he won the Northeast Harbor Road Race several times and had a marathon best of 2:29. You cannot, however, make a living winning local road races, so Westphal spent long days back on the island building homes, some of which had sculpted pools and tennis courts overlooking the ocean. He kept racing but did fewer and fewer miles after age 35.

The day we visited, Westphal drove me and Ellis down that road from the dock, pointing out about a dozen houses he had built and noting the one restaurant in town. Eventually, we reached a private road with a sign telling us to turn around. But for Westphal there aren't any private roads in Great Cranberry. He's the caretaker of 35 houses, and he seems to know everyone. If anyone is wealthy enough to have a private road, Westphal probably built the house at its end, and he's allowed to drive through. Everyone likes him. "If you do good work, you never have a problem. They can complain about the price, but if you do good work they'll be happy in the end," he says. For most of his career, he was something of a benevolent monopolist. Other carpenters would show up on the island from time to time, but, Westphal notes, "the competitors would just come and go."

The private road turns quickly into dirt and then into a kind of muddy sand. Westphal is scrunched up behind the wheel, his head still shaking rapidly from side to side, telling stories about running on the roads and the houses he's worked on.

Eventually we get to a stunning yoga studio that he built for a client. Out the left window of the car you can see Cadillac Mountain and the ridges of Acadia National Park. On the right, there's a walkway, crossable at low tide only, to tiny Crow Island. We park and navigate across the loose stones. Westphal seems like he should be unsteady, but he's not. He jumps down little ledges, and crosses pools of water. He doesn't slip on the seaweed. Eventually we reach the end of the point, looking out into the ocean. A small seal swims in the distance. He notes that he rarely falls because he has "good recovery balance."

In 2003, when he was 46, he started to feel like his left shoulder was sore all the time. Perhaps, he thought, his muscles were tight or damaged from digging so many post holes. He went to a physical therapist and then, in 2006, to a neurologist. She told him to try a drug called carbidopa-levodopa, which helps supplement dopamine, the neurotransmitter depleted in Parkinson's. When Westphal responded to the medication, it confirmed the diagnosis. Westphal didn't believe it at first. How could he have this? It was just a sore shoulder. The sore shoulder got worse, however, and, a few years later, when he was 55, his body started to shake uncontrollably.

At first, he quit running entirely. He was embarrassed by the illness and hated the way he looked when he ran on the main road. He was a carpenter: strong and steady. He didn't want everyone to stare at him and wonder. He stopped going down to the store in town because he didn't want anyone to see him spill a coffee. Gradually, though, he realized that running gave him a relief from the pressures of the diagnosis, and maybe from the physical pain too. He would tie his hands loosely together with shoestring so his left arm wouldn't flail.

He learned that if he could get moving reasonably quickly, he wouldn't wave around as much. "Once you get going," he said to me, "it's like a bike wheel."

He started to train seriously again, and he began to find a new camaraderie in the sport. He started to care less about the outcome and more about the community. People wanted to talk with him about his illness; they wanted to understand him. "There's more to running than just beating people. I realized that when I was 58," he told me.

His symptoms, though, kept getting worse. He got on a steady cycle with his medicine. Soon after taking the pill, his body would steady but his reactions would dull. He would sometimes try to counter the dullness by running. "Sometimes I get slow, and I'll just run a quarter-mile. When I start, my knees will knock together. But by the time I get back, I'll be running naturally, and the slowness will be gone." When the pill wore off, his body would start to flail but his mind would be more alert. He needs to be in different states to do different tasks. When his mind is dulled, he can't really drive. His face becomes expressionless. When his body is flailing, he can't pull up his pants. He says that he doesn't expect Parkinson's to decrease his life expectancy, unless he succumbs to a peculiar but genuine fear: suffocating while putting on a sweatshirt.

He learned to titrate his pills before a long run or a race. He would take one pill half an hour before the race, and then another two and a half hours in. So many things can go wrong when you have Parkinson's, so he always makes sure to have friends with him as wingmen in every race. After the diagnosis, he ran seven marathons, including two on Cranberry Island organized by Allen. Both times, he fell down not far from the finish. In the first race, people on the sidelines were worried he wouldn't get up. But he did, and then he stumbled forward to earn a time that qualified him for entry into the Boston Marathon. In most of his recent marathons, he finished in the top three in his age group.

When I visited him that summer, his symptoms had continued to worsen, and he could no longer work with his hands. He still checked on houses, though, and he managed a construction business. His wife was suffering through chemotherapy for a brain tumor, so he was taking care of her too. As Ellis and I sat on the end of the beach with him, I asked him what Parkinson's had taught him. "Humility," he said. People now stare at him and little girls seeing him for the first time ask him why he's dancing. "Because I love to dance," he'll say, before watching their parents shush them away. "You just have to learn to cope with it and to tie your shoes twice," he says. "You have to learn to pull your pants up and put your shirt on. And you have to learn how to ask for help from complete strangers."

Two years later, I visited him again. Now, he was living on the mainland, helping to take care of Jennifer; her condition had gotten much worse, and she couldn't get on and off the boat. Westphal was better in some ways: a procedure called deep brain stimulation had eliminated his problems with movement, but he could no longer run. He tries every now and then to do it, even if just for a mile. But he can't keep his balance. If there's even a slight downhill, he'll fall. Having Parkinson's means coping with a process of losing one ability after another. "I wanted to run as long as I could," he says wistfully. "I knew things were dropping from my life. I figured I'd keep running as long as I could. And I did."

CHAPTER 14

I Wanted to Run a Loop

> *As I got older it hit me harder; Dr. Freud says the most important day in a man's life is the death of his father. Mozart was thus freed up to write* **Don Giovanni** *when his grasping credit-claiming dad died. It took me a while to realize I hadn't allowed myself to excel athletically until he was gone.*
>
> —W. SCOTT THOMPSON, UNPUBLISHED MEMOIR

THERE ARE FOUR STATES OF RUNNING THAT I CONSIDER BLISS. THE first is meditation: you're running up a mountain or crossing a ridge. You're alone, studying the trees or the sky. Your feet land quietly on the soil, the leaves, the rocks. The kaleidoscope wheel of the mind slows. You don't have to be going fast, but, for me at least, it helps to be doing something hard. I couldn't reach this state if I took a gondola to the most beautiful vista in the world and started there. I can only reach it if I've run up a narrow trail, following painted marks on the trees, piles of rocks, or just the faint trace of runners and animals that have gone this route before. This is the kind of run I hope I can go on for at least another decade or two.

The second is flow. Here you're out on a road, pushing hard.

You're going fast and feeling strong, moving steadily and rhythmically. Your mind is active and fully present in the motion. It helps if the road is flat and the weather isn't great. A little bit of wind or rain adds flavor to the sport. This is the state I dream about when I start to get in shape. I know that more of these runs are behind me than ahead of me, but the places where I've done these runs are forever etched in my mind.

The third is catharsis. Something has gone wrong in the world or in your life, and you're not able to fully process it. You're not running to seek shelter; you're running because you seek the storm. Your mind is like molten metal and you have to run hard and heat everything up before you can cool into a new shape. My friend Michael Joyner of the Mayo Clinic, and a former 2:25 marathoner, told me that the most intense stage of his running life came when he was getting divorced. The way to handle the pain of his life was to go out on the track and create even more pain there.

The last state is oneness, and it's the hardest to reach. I can only get it at the end of a long race, and, usually, I don't even get it there. I'm still in control of my speed and my effort. I've calibrated things so that I know exactly how much energy I have left. I can't hear my friends on the sides of the course, and my field of vision has narrowed. Brain and body have merged entirely into one, but I'm not shutting down. This is the true bliss: when you know you've calibrated things perfectly. You're exhausted but you're still moving forward exactly the way you want to.

This last state was the one I had finally learned how to reach through my fast Boston Marathon and my 2:29 in Chicago. I craved it and wanted more. But the world was about to turn upside down.

∎

In January 2020, I traveled to Iowa to interview several of the Democratic presidential candidates for *CBS Sunday Morning*. One parenting lesson I learned from my father is to bring your children along whenever you're doing something that interests them. Ellis, at age 11, was into politics, so I took him with me everywhere, though he wisely stayed in the hotel one morning as I ran through Des Moines while the temperature hit a "feels like" of minus 10. The power went out when I was supposed to interview Joe Biden, then the underdog former vice president. He told Ellis to come and sit across from him and ask any question he wanted. "What was your favorite book as a kid?" Ellis asked Biden. It was a superb question, and I couldn't have been prouder.

There were worrying signs of a virus spreading in China, then Seattle, then Westchester. I gathered the staff of *Wired* and told them this might well be the story of their lives. We didn't know what was going to happen next, but it was possible we would never be in the middle of something so big again. We shut down the office soon thereafter. I watered my plants a little more than usual on the final day, assuming I'd be back in a couple of weeks. We packed the family up and headed to our house in the Catskills, a few hours north of New York City. We invited Danielle's parents to join us in a pandemic pod. I even packed up the philodendron. Miraculously, it was now 29 years old.

My job became managing *Wired*'s coverage of the pandemic and the fractal complexity of the country's medical response. Life outside work was simpler. There was no travel, no dinners, no commute. My social circle, and my social obligations, narrowed. Everyone in my immediate circle, at least for now, stayed healthy. Every day was now the same, which made it easier to create structures and habits. I went to bed every night between 10 and 11 and woke up every morning at 6. By 6:10, I would be out the door, connecting my watch to the stars and stumbling forward up our rocky driveway. I'd come home, cook everyone breakfast, and then get to work by 8:30. At 3 p.m., Zachary, James, and I would run outside to play soccer. We called it "La Masia" after the FC Barcelona youth academy, and the staff at *Wired* knew not to schedule anything for the next hour. I'd go back to work, we'd all have dinner, and then we'd play soccer again as the sun set.

I ran more consistently than at any other point in my life. I developed good habits and regular routines. An "Oreo cow loop" was 8 miles around a small mountain with a pasture with black-and-white cows. A "Schjeldahl loop" was 11.5 miles out on a gorgeous dirt road that eventually led me past the house of a dear friend, *The New Yorker*'s art critic Peter Schjeldahl. I marked segments all over town in the social media app Strava so that I could at least race against myself. (This raised an interesting dilemma: Is it better to run a bit slower so that your future self can experience the joy of beating your current self?) One day, I ran up and down three mountains with my friend Yung. We wrapped bandanas around our faces and stayed six feet apart. Running offered me a routine and helped me feel strong as the world came undone. Yung loved to run deep into the mountains, sometimes for almost a day at a time. He explained that he had lost his 20s to drug addiction. The pain he found deep into a long run reminded him of the pain he had felt in withdrawal. He wanted to remember that so he would never succumb to temptation again.

In the fall of 2020, I signed up for a marathon in Harrisburg, Pennsylvania. The race was on a Saturday morning, and I decided to stay safe from the virus by sleeping in my car. I worked all Friday dealing with a barrage of responses and tips that I had received after writing a story for *Wired* on a hiker known as "Mostly Harmless," who had died mysteriously in Florida after hiking on the Appalachian Trail. Then I headed down to the small island in the Susquehanna River, just west of the city, where the race would start. I parked near a boat ramp and a broken streetlight. I pulled down the back seat in the hatchback, unrolled a sleeping bag, and curled awkwardly inside. At 1 A.M., a group of twentysomethings screeched into the lot. For reasons I couldn't quite understand, they put one car between two large plastic barricades and revved the engine over and over again while a man and a woman sang the jingle, "Like a good neighbor, State Farm is there." An hour or so later, they mercifully disappeared.

I woke up at sunrise and headed over to the start. The course was flat and beautiful, following a river. I started off running exactly the pace I wanted. But about 12 miles in, as the course rounded a corner onto a secluded city path, I felt a shooting pain in my abdomen. It was probably only a few seconds before I stopped to walk. It was too much. I tried to run. It hurt. I walked. I tried again. And then I gave up. The course was, mercifully, a big loop, so I wasn't far from my car. I walked back to it holding my side and texted Danielle. She was surprised to have a text come in so soon. She called immediately. "It's a really hard sport," she said.

I drove home in agony wondering, as most runners do with all injuries, whether it would be gone the next day or whether it would end my running career. There's a certain warm satisfaction that comes with both thoughts. Back at my laptop, I did the natural thing of diagnosing myself via Reddit and LetsRun.com, which of course led to the conclusion that I would likely be in a wheelchair for the rest of my life. But the pain went away, and I was back running by the middle of the next week. I scheduled a time to jog with Julia Lucas. When we met, I told her what had happened. We were standing near the statue of John F. Kennedy in the inner island of Grand Army Plaza. She listened carefully to my tale of woe. Then she pushed her finger into my abdomen, precisely where it had hurt. "Is this it?" she asked. I jumped back a little and responded that, indeed, it was. She then asked, "Did you sleep oddly the night before? Maybe in a car?" I had, she diagnosed, injured my psoas muscle, and I would be fine.

Two weeks later, I decided that I would just run a marathon by myself: covering more than 13 loops around a two-mile course in Prospect Park. So that Sunday, at 6 A.M., I walked up to the park. Finley lived nearby and was waiting for me. I marked a little starting line at Grand Army Plaza and stretched myself out. There wasn't a gun or fanfare or even nerves. I just bolted off with my friend Jack, who planned to run 20 miles. I know every little hill, and almost every little drainage grate, on the loop. Marathons are supposed to be different: your body is primed and tapered, people are cheering, you're surrounded by others doing pretty much the same thing. But I had turned it all inside out. Now I was running on a road I run on damn near every day; I was passing lots of runners, but they weren't racing. I had either flattened everything special about the marathon or heightened everything about my daily run. Either way, I just settled in, watched my heart rate, and tried to breathe. Finley trailed along on a bicycle, a little behind or a little ahead, just keeping an eye on things. He's 6'5", but he was riding a bike owned by his then girlfriend, who's 5'4".

I had told Jack that I wanted to run under 2:40, which meant roughly a 6:07 pace. But we ran the first mile in 5:59 and the second in 6:02. We passed the half in 1:18:10. Each loop, the Bartel-Pritchard farmers market in the southwest corner of the park got a little fuller, with more apples, pastries, and greens appearing every 12 minutes as Jack and I hustled by. I salivated a bit at the sourdough.

I still wasn't pushing it, though. I was just running hard, watching my heart rate creep up slowly and my legs feel slightly heavier. I could feel some pain, but I couldn't localize it. I tried to understand exactly why my legs were heavy: Were the muscles tearing? And where was the pain, whatever it was, exactly? The fatigue stretched more or less from my calves up to the top of my glutes. At 25 miles, the familiar little demon behind my ear told me to drop out. I had done a good workout, and really this was just a workout. Who cared? I pushed him aside and tried to accelerate into the turns. I persevered through my last passage through the farmers market, now breathing hard with my heart rate in the 150s, near my max.

In the last mile, I tried to accelerate but something held me back. Too many strange things hurt in too many strange places. Then, suddenly, as I rounded the last curve into the park, all those strange pains vanished. I was pushing myself close to my absolute limits, and now it seemed as though my brain had finally decided I wasn't going to die. It would let me do what my body wanted for the last bit. I was confirming the Central Governor Model theory of fatigue. I sprinted down the final hill and finished in 2:35.

I walked home shaking and freezing. I lay on the floor, covered in a blanket, while Ellis brought the space heater nearby. I couldn't eat, I couldn't drink, I could barely see. It was like my entire body had been turned off. I couldn't stretch. Ellis was confused at why I seemed so broken, and I explained that a 100-percent effort is very different from a 95-percent or even a 98-percent effort. I can run a hard workout and then go out and play soccer with my boys. But I had crossed some breaking point that morning. He turned on the movie *Lincoln* and we watched Daniel Day-Lewis slowly try to win the votes for the Thirteenth Amendment. Afterward, Ellis said, "I'm definitely not going to be a distance runner when I grow up." I noted that he had exactly predicted what my time would be in this race and wondered what he thought the next one would be. "3:10," he answered.

When I was running, Zachary and James had been off in Long Island at soccer games. But the next day, I went for a walk in Prospect Park with a prospective colleague. I was in the final stages of negotiating a new job as CEO of *The Atlantic*. I had become convinced that my greatest skill in journalism wasn't writing or editing: it was figuring out creative business models to support others doing that work. This was a chance to fully test that hypothesis at a publication I had read since I was a child. Most of the negotiations had happened via Zoom because of the pandemic, but today we decided to talk while out on a stroll. As we passed across a trail that cut through the center of the park, I saw a little figure in a Barcelona uniform and a blue coat come jogging along next to a slightly older kid on a bike. It was James, then six years old, with a friend who lived next door. "What are you doing? I asked. "I wanted to run a loop," he said.

I had, it seemed, by the very same race encouraged one child to become a runner and another to pledge he would avoid the sport forever.

■

The last time I ran with my father was probably around the year 2001. At the time, I was living with him in Washington, D.C., in his beautiful, impractical brick house just off Rock Creek Park. I was working 90 to 100 hours a week at *The Washington Monthly*, and I wasn't finding much time to run. But every now and then we would put on our sneakers and head down Broad Branch Road to a little paved path above the creek. After a bit more than two miles, we'd reach the entrance to the National Zoo and turn right. We'd pass by the Reptile House. We'd hear exotic birds screeching and take in the whiff of elephant dung. Eventually, we'd reach Connecticut Avenue and the heart of the neighborhood known as Cleveland Park. We would turn right, run north, and head home.

At some point we surely crossed paths with a small woman with blue eyes, freckles, and long reddish-brown hair. She was in her mid-40s then, halfway between my father's and my ages, and she ran with a light step, more like a gazelle than a cheetah. Her favorite loop included most of the one my father and I ran: she'd go down from Connecticut Avenue, through the zoo, and up the roads by the creek. But then she'd just keep going into Maryland. Eventually, she'd loop back and head down Connecticut Avenue. We were running a four-mile square, and she was running a 20- or 30-mile rectangle that included the square. She lived near the gift store she owned called Transcendence-

Perfection-Bliss of the Beyond. I passed it almost every day but never went in.

I doubt we would have noticed her. You pass a lot of people when you run, and my mind then was on work, work, work. When we ran, I would ask my father about my articles and I'd test out headlines on him. We'd talk about power in Washington, my career, his grievances, and who might come to the next dinner party we were going to host.

I can imagine us now. Me with longish hair and tired eyes, 20 or 30 pounds heavier than I am today. I'm running in bulky Saucony shoes and wearing a worn, blue political T-shirt from my college days with the Earth upside down and the words "Student Environmental Action Coalition" written across it. He's balding and somewhat disheveled in a Lacoste shirt with an alligator above the chest and a tear at the armpit. He's wearing dress socks pulled high that don't quite match. He's in New Balance shoes that he's had for a decade but misplaced for years at a time. I'm talking about something stressful at work. We're in the sweltering D.C. humidity, passing under the tulip trees and expecting a thunderstorm. Little packs of tiny gnats hover every few hundred feet, right about head height. Then the quiet, unassuming wisp of a woman crosses by. She's closed the gift store and put on her shoes. She's breathing steadily and listening to the sound of the creek. Her eyes are open in a way that ours are not. She has tried to turn off her mind so she can listen to her heart. She's wearing a light T-shirt that declares "Sri Chinmoy Marathon Team." Her name is Suprabha Beckjord, and she is the greatest ultramarathoner in the world.

CHAPTER 15

Suprabha Beckjord

If you make your speed-flow
Very fast,
And your concentration-power
Very penetrating,
Then daily you can accomplish
So many things.

—SRI CHINMOY

THE FIRST TIME SUPRABHA BECKJORD WENT RUNNING, SHE MEASURED her progress in telephone poles. It was the late 1970s, and she had just graduated from Bennington College. She was painting and living in a family house near the ocean in Sorrento, Maine. She read a book by a guru from India named Sri Chinmoy who believed that running could serve as a pathway for spiritual growth. Beckjord was drawn to the idea, so she laced her shoes, went out on the tiny, quiet road by her house, and ran to the third telephone pole off in the distance. Another day, she ran to the fourth one. Eventually she wrote to Chinmoy, who welcomed her into his group. As he did for many of his several thousand disciples, he gave her a new first name. She had grown up as "Amy" but now she would be "Suprabha," which means "radiant" and "beautiful light."

Chinmoy Kumar Ghose was born in India in 1931 and orphaned at the age of 12. He entered an ashram, where he began an intensive study of meditation and spirituality. His ashram taught that the dogged pursuit of excellence in sports was a way to reconstruct both mind and body. In 1964, he flew to New York City and moved to Greenwich Village. Chinmoy was compassionate and charismatic, and he combined ideas that were in vogue, like spirituality, with ones that were not, like celibacy. He fused an Eastern mysticism with a deeply American immigrant hustle. He understood the rubrics of both eternal life and *The Pat Collins Show*. By 1970, he was leading regular meditation sessions at the United Nations. He led them, too, at the start of the New York City Marathon. The great guitarist John McLaughlin became a follower. Sri Chinmoy began to play the flute and he started to paint. He was said to sleep just 90 minutes a night, giving him plenty of time to practice both.

In the mid-seventies, Chinmoy began to formulate his philosophy of running. He proposed that one way to transcend the world that we are in was to push our feet into the ground and absorb the light from the sky. Running, done properly, was meditation and a way to connect to a higher reality. He founded what he called the Sri Chinmoy Marathon Team. Runners, he believed, should try their hardest and seek to do better each time. They should seek to understand the complex intersection of discipline, surrender, and devotion. He wanted his followers to test their limits and compete, but he was teaching competition in the service of self-awareness, not the other way around. "From start to finish / I run / Only to be closer to God," he wrote.

Beckjord is about 5'3" and lean as a sandpiper. She's quiet and gentle and exudes kindness in a way that reflects her name. She has light freckles and ties her hair back in a bun. Around the time she began studying with Chinmoy, she opened the store on Connecticut Avenue in Washington, close to my father's house. Chinmoy instructed her to name it "Transcendence-Perfection-Bliss of the Beyond," which probably would not have won a McKinsey branding exercise. When not studying under Chinmoy, she'd work there, selling cards and stuffed animals and playing the guru's music to customers. I must have gone by it several hundred times when I lived in Washington, but I didn't go in until I was in my 40s. When I first went in to talk with her, I felt as though I was in the presence of a saint.

Once Beckjord was accepted into the group, she began to pray and meditate intensely. This, she said, developed her willpower and, in turn, endurance. In January 1980, she traveled with Sri Chinmoy up to Burlington, Vermont, where he was giving a concert. After the performance, he declared that his followers should stage what he called an "Inspiration Marathon" in the subfreezing weather at 6 A.M. the next day. Beckjord thus entered and finished her first race: 26.2 miles in the blistering wind. She loved it.

From then on, Beckjord started to run, and run, and run. Chinmoy plotted out ever more extreme challenges for his followers, and the longer the run, the more Beckjord wanted to do it. It wasn't long before she was measuring her runs in sunrises, not telephone poles. She ran a five-day race comprised of loops around New York's Flushing Meadows Corona Park, and then a seven-day race. She ran 1,300 miles in 18 days. She almost always beat all the other women. She's spiritual and sweet—with the competitive spirit of Kobe Bryant.

Chinmoy's birthday was August 27, and he decided, in 1996, to start a 2,700-mile race, which would make it by far the longest in the world. The course would be a single block in Queens, around Thomas A. Edison Career and Technical Education High School, and abutting the Grand Central Parkway. Chinmoy lived nearby and picked it precisely for its normalcy. Each loop would be about half a mile around a playground, a soccer field, and the school. Such a course made the logistics easier. It's roughly 2,700 miles from San Francisco to New York, and you could organize a race over the route. But the runners wouldn't know where to sleep or eat, and sometimes they'd get lost. Their minds might also drift to the vistas of the Rockies or the joy of crossing the Mississippi. In this new race, the runners would just loop around the gritty park again and again. The race combined the epic and the mundane.

That first year, Beckjord was the only woman to finish the race, and thus the winner. The next year, Chinmoy decided to match the distance to the year of his birth, making it 3,100 miles. Beckjord entered and won again. She would complete the race, and win the women's category, the next 13 years in a row. In total, she ran roughly 43,000 miles around that block in Queens, the equivalent of running one and a half times around the Earth. During the rest of the year, she would go back to Connecticut Avenue and train just like a normal person: 45 minutes a day with a long run on the weekends.

The 3,100-mile race was given particular rules. Runners would start each day at 6 A.M. with a single minute of meditation. Then they would begin to race. At midnight, they had to go rest. One day they would circle the block clockwise; the next day they'd change direction. When you run that much, you'll end up bent like a banana if your left shoulder is always to the curve. A runner once had to leave the race when his visa expired. Most of the people in the neighborhood admired the runners; some were confused. "Those are the fucking craziest people," Tony Ruiz, who lives nearby, once told me.

Beckjord allowed herself a short break, of about 15 minutes, in the early afternoon, and then another similar one at about 5 P.M. The goal was to finish in 52 days or faster, which meant a minimum of 60 miles a day. She liked it when she could complete the mileage she needed by 10:30 or 11 P.M. Sri Chinmoy believed that one could train oneself to recover in a short period of time. Sleeping three hours, if done with focus and intentionality, could heal the body as much as sleeping eight. Beckjord, after running 60 miles, liked to get at least five hours of rest before she rose, meditated, and headed to the course to do it again.

The race began in the summer, and she ran through lightning storms, pouring rain, and oppressive heat. On scorching days, she'd put her legs and shoes into a big plastic bag and then lower herself into a bucket of ice. She regularly got blisters the size of cherries. She slathered on baking soda to help prevent rashes. One year, she lost five toenails; a friend suggested that she should get a half-price pedicure. Friends would come to the course and give her food that she would eat as she ran. She estimates that she took in about 10,000 calories a day. Spectators watched and cheered, often unaware of who was ahead, who was behind, or even who was running. Chinmoy had created the world's longest race, and it didn't look like a race at all.

Beckjord most liked to run in the early mornings when it was cool and in the evenings when it was quiet. The days were louder, with men playing pickup basketball and handball on the high school courts. One day a woman on a bench sang a beautiful rendition of "Amazing Grace." Meanwhile, Beckjord just kept circling around. "It isn't a real race," one of the competitors said, "unless you have to get your hair cut in the middle of it."

When she would tire, she would focus on her breath. She would try to imagine that she was a six- or seven-year-old child. She would try to feel joy that would pass through the earth and bring joy to someone on the far side of the world. Chinmoy had once written, "The body's capacity and the soul's capacity, the body's speed and the soul's speed, go together. The outer running reminds us of something higher and deeper—the soul—which is running along Eternity's Road."

Beckjord told me that she smiles when she's in pain. It helps her and it helps the other runners in the race. She learned that from Chinmoy, but it also squares with the research. When cyclists are shown images of smiling faces while they ride, their endurance improves. Eliud Kipchoge knows this too: when you watch him run a race, he looks effortless and smooth. The only way you can tell he's in pain is when a broad smile appears on his face.

Beckjord learned to meditate by listening to the sounds of the cars on the Grand Central Parkway. She would turn the hum of their motors into the sound "om." She would watch and track little flowers growing up on the side of the course. Sometimes, she would imagine that she was running on a country road or back counting lampposts. She didn't count laps or miles. "The surface that you run on is solid concrete," she says. "When you're running around hour after hour, you feel like the ground you're striking against is striking your mind. You start thinking, *This is so bad: I have to run sixty miles every day.* But it's the mind counting. It can torture you. You have to let it go." She would allow herself to think about the end only when she reached 200 miles to go. Then, with 100 miles to go, she started to think of it as her victory lap. "Then you were only going to have one of each number from that point."

The race was, to Beckjord, "a pilgrimage." When she was running, she would think that the effort was her little contribution to human progress. She'd do it for two months and then begin the gradual transition back to regular life, which wasn't always simple. She hadn't touched money or bought anything for two months. Her life had been distilled to its essence: run, eat, sleep, repeat. Now, back in Washington, she had employees and inventory to manage in her store. People weren't helping with her food. One day, shortly after finishing, at a friend's apartment by herself, she decided to make a smoothie. She carefully placed everything in the blender and pressed the start button. Juice sprayed everywhere. She had forgotten to put the top on.

In 2010 she decided that her body couldn't do it anymore. She came to the course that year and watched the runners get ready to start the first morning. She felt so compelled to head out with them that she had to hug a tree and hold on tight. She watched, wistfully, as they passed the soccer field. She saw the traffic on the Grand Central Parkway, heading to LaGuardia, JFK, the Upper East Side, Connecticut, New Jersey. There are seasons in life, and now she knew that it was time to rest.

The first time I went to watch the race was in the early fall of 2023. The September leaves were just starting to drift down and accumulate on the sidewalk. Yellow tape covered every little bump in the concrete, alerting the runners as they navigated evening darkness or morning delirium. At what's called base camp, by the starting line, volunteers had set up tents and tables. They handed out food and applauded every time a runner completed a loop. I came back five or six times and would occasionally run loops with different runners. They often wanted to know what was happening in the world; in mid-October, I explained to one of them that war had broken out the week before between Hamas and Israel.

One day, James and I were at the course watching and talking with the runners. A familiar face appeared on the sidelines. Beckjord had taken a day off from the store and come to Queens to cheer the runners on. James and I joined her to run a lap. She took us to a beautiful pine tree on one of the corners of the course. It was, she said, her favorite spot. She spoke wistfully about her summers of running: "My life is so complex now. Back then, all I had to do is go around in circles."

CHAPTER 16

A Labrador in a Race for Wolves

I think about many things during the week, seldom about my father, but when I sit down to do something so serious as to write about my thoughts, I can only write about him.
—W. SCOTT THOMPSON, DIARY ENTRY, MARCH 31, 1974

FOR YEARS, I STUCK TO MARATHONS. IN 2021, THOUGH, I DECIDED TO TRY something at least a touch longer. My friend Josh Cox was then the agent to one of my running idols, the Olympian Desiree Linden. She had spent the period of Covid lockdowns training like she had lost a bet while playing beer pong. In October 2020, she had run one mile on the first day of the month, two on the second, and so on, until she ran 31 miles on the 31st. Now, Cox told me, she was going to try to set the world record in the 50K, a distance just over 31 miles. Would I be interested in helping to pace her? The women's world record of 3:07 was just one minute off the men's American record in my age group. Most of the major marathons were still canceled. I said I was in.

Technically, an "ultramarathon" is any race longer than a marathon, and a 50K perhaps shouldn't count. It's like someone who boasts of wanting to see the world beyond America—and then goes to Toronto. But to me, it was still an unknown frontier. The age-group record was held by Michael Wardian, a legend of ultrarunning who had won the Delaware Marathon when I had run it in 2005. Finley made me a schedule that wasn't much different from what I had used before my breakthrough race in Chicago a year and a half before. My long runs got a little longer. My tempo intervals stretched out a little farther. The complexity increased. One day, I ran five miles at roughly my marathon pace; I rested for five minutes and then ran six half-miles at my half-marathon pace. In the middle of the training, I started my new job as CEO of *The Atlantic*. I took one week off between jobs, during which I managed to get in a particularly grueling workout.

The race was scheduled for early April, but the exact day wouldn't be locked in until the very end. Cox had selected a flat course in Oregon, where he knew the weather would be cool. He'd blocked out a couple of days, and we'd run whenever conditions seemed best. He couldn't have too many people in the race because Covid was still a threat. As the race approached, Linden's goal got more ambitious. She didn't just want the record; she wanted to break 3 hours. This meant that I'd be useless as a pacer; she needed someone quicker. Josh told me to come anyway. I'd be behind her, but I could try to run the fastest time by a man over 45.

The night before the race, I sat in my hotel room in Eugene and tried to work through my normal pre-race routine. I laid out my uniform: Nike half-tights and my paper-thin green singlet with *Wired* emblazoned on the back. I ate a pre-race dinner of salted bread with almond butter and a beet salad. I drank cup after cup of water, filled at the bathroom sink. I clipped my toenails, shaved the tiny hairs off the tops of my feet, and scraped all the dirt off my racing shoes. Maybe I could save one second by doing all this; maybe I'd need that second; maybe the simple act would just give me a little motivation at the end. I lay flat on my back on the hotel bed, looked upward, and tried to visualize the course and how I would move through it. I would do this, I planned, until I fell asleep.

Something was scaring me, though. I was worried about something more than the possibility of failure and something less than the possibility of death. I didn't know how this lean, imperfect body that I inhabited could cross that much ground at such a pace. I texted Brett Kirby, the Nike sports scientist, and asked him what I should do late in the race. Kirby was smart enough to know that I wasn't really texting him about what to do late in the race. What you are about to do, he said, is hard. Don't focus on that. Focus on something that you've done before that's harder. Change it, he suggested, to "less than something else bigger." I began to think about the workouts I had done, on little sleep and on smoggy streets, at speeds much faster than I would have to run the next day. I thought about the Escarpment Run. I sent him another note asking why, when drafting, it's useful to have runners behind you as well as ahead of you. He explained that every runner creates a little air bubble that can actually give a slight push to the runner ahead. I smiled and drifted off to sleep.

The next morning, Finley drove me out to the start. He had brought a bicycle so that he could accompany me. I warmed up in the parking lot and marveled at the running royalty who had shown up for this tiny race on a cold day in April on the Row

River. One of the pacers was Peter Bromka, a 2:19 marathoner and a terrific writer. The race director was Ian Dobson, Julia Lucas's ex-husband. He had been a star at Stanford and then an Olympian. Ryan Hall, the fastest American marathoner of all time, was there too. He had taken up weightlifting and transformed himself from a string bean to a baked potato. He told me that he wanted to become the first person to deadlift 500 pounds and then run a 5-minute mile. Linden was warming up with her pacer, Charlie Lawrence, a qualifier for the Olympic Trials marathon. She wore red sunglasses and a fluorescent yellow Brooks singlet. She looked ripped and ready. She's 5'1" and 100 pounds of muscle: a tiny tactical missile with a ponytail.

We lined up, many of us wearing face coverings that we would pull down after the crowded start. I didn't want to run alone, so I fell in behind a little group that included Chirine Njeim, a Lebanese runner who had competed in three winter Olympics in alpine skiing and was now trying to qualify for her second summer Olympics in the marathon. Hall was coaching Njeim, and he led her on a bike. She wanted music, so another biker was carrying a boom box. About three miles in, I made my best decision of the race. We were running 5:53s, only four seconds faster than my goal pace, but something felt wrong. I slowed and told Finley that I was going to leave this little pack. When I look back, I can remember the moment and the choice. But I can't explain precisely what I felt or how I knew. I could just tell that my body was working a little too hard for the task ahead.

The course was on a narrow bike path through a forest of ponderosa pines. It was flat, quiet, and cool, just the conditions you need to run fast. Cox had called it a "no excuses" day. I concentrated on my mantras: right foot, left foot, right foot, and steadied my pace as I've never steadied it before. I felt strong, as though I was running through an Escher staircase with a very faint downward slope. We traveled 6.5 miles straight out, and then looped around a pylon and went back. This meant that, four times, I passed Linden going the other direction. "Go, Des," I'd shout. "Go, Nick," she'd respond.

I passed 10 miles in 59:25 and then ran the next 10 in 59:21. I passed Njeim and the boom box and pulled myself back into the quiet. Finley pedaled a little bit ahead, saying almost nothing. He knew that I was in control. I tried to concentrate on him and the road. Whenever we passed the tall trees, I would look up and try to draw energy from them. I'd think of how old they were and all the wind and sunlight that had passed through them. I'd ask for some of that strength to keep pushing me forward.

After two full loops, I crossed the marathon line and turned around again. This time the pylon would be just 2.5 miles away. Linden came scorching by for the final time. She looked like a Corvette ZL1 driving south while I felt like a Honda Odyssey chugging north. "Go, Des!" "Go, Nick!" My third 10-mile block was 59:27. Soon the finish was in sight. I sprinted. Linden had already broken the tape, set a world record, and then wandered off to the side to puke. I was two minutes ahead of the old record for my age group, so Cox pulled out the tape again. I surged toward it, racing some runner in the future who will be trying to beat my time. My mind had narrowed completely: like I was running through a straw just barely wide enough for me to finish. I crossed the finish in 3:04:36.

Twenty-eight years before, on the track in Deerfield, Massachusetts, I had run in a primal way, screaming inside and giving it everything a young man could. I crossed the line and then the lights went out. It was a 9-minute race and I was one teenager chasing another. Now I was 45, I'd been running for three hours, and I was chasing a time. But in those last moments of the race, I remembered that green track 28 years before. When we're teenagers, we're pulled by instinct and our emotions are thunderstorms that sweep away hillsides inside our minds. Now my emotions were those of an older man: a steady rain that formed a river pushing relentlessly forward. I had planned, prepared, and executed. I had used the skills I had learned in a lifetime of running and a lifetime of focused work to run the best race of my life. I didn't scream inside like I had on the Deerfield track, but that doesn't mean I didn't feel as intensely. Right after I crossed the line, I started to wobble and then I toppled over.

Eventually I steadied myself and gave Finley a big hug. Then I stumbled over to congratulate Des. I changed from my singlet into a black Boston Bruins T-shirt. Tradition holds that after setting a record, you should drink champagne out of your running shoes. It was a Brooks event, and I had run in Nikes. Des's husband asked whether I would like to drink out of his running shoes. I was committed to the project but not so much that I would take down a shot of my new friend's toe sweat. I held my hand over the Nike swoosh as I poured champagne down my own shoes.

My new *Atlantic* colleagues mostly learned about the race from Twitter. Many of them had some sense that I was a runner, but they didn't know the depth of my passion. I was a little proud, naturally, but also worried. Would they see this sport as a frivolous distraction from my serious new job? *The Atlantic* was founded in 1857 by Ralph Waldo Emerson, Harriet Beecher Stowe, Oliver Wendell Holmes Sr., and other great trinomial luminaries of the nineteenth century to try to save American democracy in the years before the Civil War. The magazine had thrived, for the most part, for 150 years. But the company had very publicly laid off 20 percent of its employees six months before I was hired. Should the skinny new CEO really be running 50Ks in a green singlet in Lane County, Oregon? Shouldn't he perhaps be meeting with advertisers in New York?

This was a variation on a common worry of mine: Does my running detract from my family and my work? Every now and then, I think I should take all my carbon-plated racing shoes and lock them in the attic. Running can be selfish and a waste of time. It wears out the skin and possibly the heart. I couldn't be the perfect parent, or the perfect CEO, even if I had 25 hours in a day. How can I possibly hope to be so if I only really have 23?

But that thought passes. Running has become part of my day where I disconnect from screens and let my mind drift usefully and turn over problems. It encourages simple habits—healthy sleep, healthy eating, moderate drinking—that help as much at 8 A.M. meetings as they do at 6 A.M. runs. It taught me to have total trust in the compound interest gained by steady day-by-day work. I got fast by running hard, consistently, and wasting very little time worrying about how ambitious my goals were. I had learned that time spent fretting about a task is almost always better spent doing the task. I had also succeeded because I had learned, through practice, how to stay calm under stress. I had saved my race by backing off early when the pace was ever-so-slightly too fast. I had just steadily run mile after mile, right up to my physical limit. I had learned this way of modulating effort through intense office work and intense running.

There were some deeper lessons too. To improve at running, you have to make yourself uncomfortable and push yourself to go at speeds that seem too fast. You need, from time to time, to move out into the "lane of high hopes." The same is true in a complicated job. I had learned that our minds create limits for us when we're afraid of failure, not because it's actually time to slow or stop. Which had done more to shape my mind: running or work? I don't know. But I do think that those two parts of my life are now deeply intertwined.

My record was a footnote. I had run a slightly obscure distance at a slightly obscure age. Half the people in that Oregon parking lot had done something more impressive at some point in their running careers. Still, I had done something faster than anyone recorded had done it before. The man whose record I had broken was a true legend of the sport. I had done something that showed I was strong at an age when so many men worry about feeling weak. A few months after I set the record, I told James that I was worried that Wardian would run faster and get it back. "Then I won't get to brag about you anymore," he said in his sweet seven-year-old voice. "And then you'll have to do it again," said Ellis.

■

After drinking the champagne out of my shoe in Oregon, I stalled out for a spell. Finley was too busy with about four new jobs to continue to manage my freelance efforts, so I just took his old Google Docs and did everything the same on my own. But training is not a math equation. The same sum of workouts did not equal the same result. I ran the Chicago Marathon the next fall in 2:37, then the Boston Marathon in 2:37, then the London Marathon in 2:35. These were objectively excellent times, but I needed something new. When you get too comfortable with anything, you stagnate. I consulted my children about all the possible next goals: running steady marathons, moving to pure mountain races, or trying to set another record at a new distance. The consensus was clear. My marathons were now boring. Setting another record would be cool.

I decided to try for the American age-group record in the 50-miler. It meant running for a bit more than five and a half hours at roughly 6:40 pace. That sounded hard, but intriguing. I entered the Tunnel Hill 50-Mile, a November race on hard-packed dirt in Vienna, Illinois, right by the Kentucky border. It's farm country, whiskey country, coal country. I chose the race because, counter to its name, it's not very hilly. Most 50-milers go up mountains or across rivers. Ultrarunners generally don't care about time; they're just trying to finish what they start. But when they want a fast time, they often come to Tunnel Hill, which hosts a 50-mile and a 100-mile race on the same day. The women's 100-mile world record was set on this course in 2017 by Camille Herron, who was born with a twist in her right femur and who runs with a motion that looks like she's cross-country skiing. Three years later, Zack Beavin, a young Kentuckian, had come to Tunnel Hill and run the fourth-fastest time of any American ever. I saw that Beavin coached over email. I wrote to him and signed him up.

There are lots of physiological differences between running 50 miles and running 26 or even 31. In a marathon, you burn almost entirely glycogen, particularly if you plan your nutrition right. In a 50-miler, your body becomes a metabolic omnivore—devouring glycogen, proteins, and fats—so you have to train your body to be efficient in this process and you need to train your gut to take in more food than you normally would. You can reach states of dehydration and energy depletion that you don't get near in a marathon. You have to deal, too, with different kinds of muscle soreness and breakdown. More important, there's a kind of deep mental fatigue that makes your mind feel like it's wrapped in steel wool. Marathon runners get tired and miserable, but they rarely get so disoriented and exhausted that they have to step off the course, lay their heads in the moss, and take a nap. Marathons are also generally linear: you run the same speed the whole way; or you run slower and slower after a certain point. Ultramarathons, as I would eventually learn, don't work that way. You can run fast and then slow and then fast again.

Beavin didn't want me to train much differently than I do for my marathons. He suggested I do a little bit less speed and some more intense long runs. He also wanted me to spend a lot of time running at my goal pace of 6:40. That's an unfamiliar zone for me. It's too slow for my workouts and far too fast for my easy days. So Beavin had me add into my routine 30- to 36-mile "Quality Long Runs," in which I would run some 6:10 miles early and then close with a long block of miles at 6:40. Beavin wanted that pace to feel familiar.

The day before the Tunnel Hill race, I flew to Nashville and rented a car. "Is this business or pleasure?" the man at the rental car pickup asked. I told him I wasn't sure. Then I drove a few hours to the pre-race pasta dinner at the local high school, where I sat next to an older man in a blue shirt. When I asked him which race he was going to do, he told me he was going to do "the hundred-miler." "At my age, you have to go for it," he added. I asked, "How old are you?" "Seventy-three," he responded. Running these distances, he said, was better than going to a psychotherapist. The man sitting across from him, likely in his 50s, nodded. "Yes, I tell my wife that the reason I haven't had a midlife crisis is because I do this. Would you rather that I got a blonde and a convertible?" A grumpy spouse might have called him out for what's called a false choice. A savvy spouse would just hand him a headlamp.

The next morning, I woke up in my Airbnb near the course, made a pot of coffee, studied the map, and organized all my gear. The key to preparation is to master the details and avoid the unexpected. Then I opened the wooden front door and was confronted with the unexpected. Contrary to the forecast, the sky had dumped snow during the night, and it was still coming down. I shuffled to the car, turned the heat on high, and wondered what the hell I was doing. I had racing shoes with no grip, thin socks, and half-tights.

Still, the race started perfectly. I stuck right with another runner, Ford McElroy, as we traversed the parking lot and then headed out on the trail. We stayed precisely on 6:40 pace and chatted about normal race banalities: the cold, the food, the speed. We had both over-hydrated, but I had, over time, trained myself to be able to pee while I ran and Ford had not. This meant that about every four miles, he would pull off, I'd slow slightly, and then he'd hustle back up. The trail was gorgeous: packed gravel, covered by light snow, stretching for what looked like miles into the distance. I felt like I was running into Monet's Snowy Road.

The miles went by smoothly. Ford and I passed through 26.2 miles in 2:54, exactly on target. It was right about then that Ford and I both noted that we weren't feeling tired, but we were feeling something that wasn't good. A little unwanted heaviness had set into my legs. At about mile 31, I reached into a pocket on my water bottle to get a gel. It was jammed in, and I had to take my glove off. My hand slipped and the gel dropped. I reached down and soon I was sprawling in the snow on a bridge, my ankle turned. I got up, but now I was cold and wet, with a hurt ankle. Ford was disappearing in the distance. Everything unraveled quickly. My left Achilles tendon started to hurt. Then my knee. I felt like I was going to throw up. I slowed to about seven minutes a mile and then eight.

I tried that impossible runner's calculation: Am I in pain because I'm tired or because I'm hurt? I couldn't quite tell. I was clearly a little bit of both. I also wondered whether this was just a reaction to a goal slipping away. I noticed, though, that most of the pain was dissipating except for in one place. My knee felt OK. My ankle felt OK. But something was definitely wrong with my Achilles. I shuffled along until the next aid station, at mile 37. There, cold and miserable, I pulled off to the side. I sat by a space heater in a tent and put my head in my hands. Volunteers offered me hot soup, peanut butter bars, and blankets. I had tried so hard and worked so hard. I had had a string of successes, and now I had a total failure. I sat for 10 or 15 minutes, shivering, and then started to wonder what I was doing, feeling sorry for myself here. No one else had come by. There were hundreds of runners in the race. I was, remarkably, still in third place. Shouldn't I just get back up and run?

It wasn't clear that I was injured. It wasn't clear, in fact, that I felt any worse than half the runners on the course. Ford, it turned out, had thrown up all over himself, and when I next saw him, looping back, he was shuffling and swaying side to side. He looked like he had just been excavated from an ancient ice core beneath a Danish bog. I realized that I'd been working with a marathoner's mentality: If I wasn't going to reach my time goal, what was the point of taking the risk? The ultrarunner's mentality is different. You run so that you come to this point—head in hands, shaking from the cold—and then press on. Trained ultrarunners are masters at ignoring pain and fatigue. But that day, I didn't have the courage. I was a Labrador running a race designed for wolves. I told a race official by the side that I was dropping out. The next morning, I took Ellis and Zachary on a short bike ride after lunch. We returned to the house right about when the last runners in Vienna were coming in.

I read about upcoming 50-milers and resolved to try again. Four days later, I strapped on my backpack and committed to running into work. I had dropped James at school and started to run when I realized that something was terribly wrong in my Achilles. I stopped after a couple of blocks and walked home. A doctor would soon confirm that I had wrecked it during the race; in fact, both my Achilles tendons were strained and on the verge of tearing. If the left one hadn't given out at mile 35, the right one might have given out at mile 38. It would be several months until I ran steadily again.

■

Two years later, at age 49, I started to really feel some of the effects of aging. I noticed that it took a lot longer to warm up for a run; small injuries healed much more slowly than in the past. If I tweaked a hamstring or turned an ankle playing soccer, it would take a month to recover, not the week it would have taken a decade earlier. I also simply couldn't go as fast. I could manage only a 5:50 pace in the workouts where I had run at 5:30 pace three years before. My endurance, however, seemed steadier. I was losing my speed but not my strength. So I decided to make my races longer. Thus, in August 2024 I found myself at the start line of the Twisted Branch 100K race in the Finger Lakes region of Upstate New York. This was an ultramarathon of a different, more primal type. Runners camped out in a meadow at the start and woke up at 3 A.M. We took down our tents, grabbed paper cups of coffee, and put our headlamps on. The race began at 4 A.M., two hours before sunrise. We scurried off into the woods, in tight single file. Two miles in, with 60 to go, my left foot crashed into a thick root, and I tumbled forward. I braced myself with my hands and was lucky to emerge with just a scrape.

The course passed lakes and circled horse pastures, gravel roads, rocky creeks, mountain vistas, and hills so steep you felt you could stretch your hands straight in front of you and touch the ground ahead. Mostly, though, we were grinding through narrow paths in the woods, trying not to lose track of the orange trail flags. Three of them meant a turn was coming up, two of them meant you had turned in the right direction, and one of them meant you were still going in the right direction. A stretch without any meant it was time to turn around. I carried so much water in my right hand that my arm began to ache. My goal was simple: finish before the sun went down.

About 30 miles in, I turned off the background noise in my mind. I was in about 20th place and had been racing the way I usually do: tracking my splits on my watch and keeping an eye on my heart rate. I realized that I had now been running for more time than I had ever run before—and I still had 32 miles to go. After the next hard five miles, I would still have a marathon left. My legs hurt; my abdomen hurt; I felt dizzy. I had been a last-minute addition off the waitlist. I had missed dinner because I'd stayed at the office a little longer than I should have and forgotten my sandwich in a mad dash to get on the bus to the campground. I had slept less than four hours. I had plenty of good reasons to drop out.

I paused for a second and turned off my heart-rate monitor. Then I flipped my watch to a screen where I couldn't see my pace. I thought of Suprabha and her recommendation that one should never dwell on how far one has to go. Then it will seem impossible. Instead, I tried to imagine that I was young Nick, bounding through the forests of New England. The trail sometimes looked just like the bird sanctuary at Andover. I let go of my concerns about time, pace, heart rate, cadence. I didn't worry how many miles had passed or how many there were to go. I just kept moving forward and tried to summon that feeling of Acadia National Park, of the magnolia tree at my grandparents' house, of Kinsman Mountain.

I felt lighter as I ran, and less worried. Every now and then, my watch would beep to signal that another mile had passed. Every hour or so, I would cruise into an aid station and eat whatever I felt like eating. I just kept moving forward and, remarkably, I seemed to pick up speed. I started passing other runners. A bee stung my calf; I could feel blisters the size of grapes forming on my feet; I stubbed my toes more times than I could count and more violently than I had ever done before. Now I had run 42, 46, 50 miles. At mile 52, I felt a touch of sadness that I only had 10 more miles to go. It was beautiful to run these trails without the pressure of wanting to finish in a certain time or to hold on to a specific place.

The race finishes on a steep descent down a mountain, the kind of terrain where I struggle and that can be agony on shredded quads. I could hear the party down at the finish line at Champlin Beach, with Bryan Adams blasting from the speakers. I sprinted across the last 100 meters of grass. I had come in eighth place and finished more than three hours before the sun would go down.

A few months afterward, in November 2024, I returned to Tunnel Hill. This time, I set a simple goal: I would finish the race with continuous forward motion. I would run as fast as I could, but my goal was to finish with honor; it was no longer to set the American record. I started off at 6:55 pace, about 15 seconds per mile slower than what I would need to run to set the record. And then I just kept on going. I held that pace for 20 miles, accelerated slightly, and then slowed slightly. In the final 10 miles, I looked to the trees and tried to remember the freedom I had felt at Twisted Branch. I finished with a smile and with strength, in 5:46, which meant that I had averaged exactly my goal pace. Five months later, I went even quicker in a 50-mile race in Connecticut and ran the fastest time in the world that year for anyone in my age group. It had taken several years, but I no longer felt like a Labrador. I had learned an entirely new way to run.

CHAPTER 17

More Than Anything

ME: Do you think that you and I are similar?
ZACHARY, AGE 13: I think we're very similar, actually. I really like training for soccer and getting better at a sport that I like. I don't like running, but the feeling is really rewarding when you've put your body through something extreme that you didn't want to do.
ME: Do you think you'll ever run a marathon?
ZACHARY: I think I will do it as soon as I can. I think it would be pretty cool to have run it. I think it's a very cool accomplishment. Not many people can. Eventually I will definitely be fit enough to run it.
ME: Which one do you want to run?
ZACHARY: New York City, of course.

I'VE STRUGGLED FOR YEARS WITH THE QUESTION OF INHERITANCE: what we give our children, what they reject from us, what they absorb without really knowing it. My father gave me his drive, which he in turn had been given by his father. I went to the same schools and did the same things; I took up his sport and developed a love for his music. For better or worse, I inherited what a don at Oxford once called his "absolute inexhaustibility," and also what the don described as his difficulty focusing in a single direction. I did not inherit his sexuality. I did not inherit his alcoholism, at least not yet. I pay my taxes. I fell in love with someone the same age who has never tried to drug our dog. I have yet to inherit the professional insecurities my father had in his 40s and 50s, but that may come.

I don't yet know what my children will take from me, and it doesn't seem fair to speculate. They are still too young. They have their own lives and dreams, and my objective in parenting is to try to support them as best I can in the lives they want to live. They're very different boys. I'm sure that, once they're adults, I'll be able to see the ways in which Danielle and I shaped them for good and for ill. I'm sure they'll have theories about the ways we stunted them or led them astray.

As I dug deeper into my father's life after his death, one revelation hit me again and again: he kept foisting the same burdens on me that his father had foisted on him. There was a moment of agony that haunted my father's life. His reaction in his later years wasn't to rebel against it. It was to repeat it.

My father had many frustrations with his father. But the most bitter was simply the pain of watching a man of ambition and purpose drown in alcohol. Frank spent the last 20 years of his working life moving from job to job. He drank to mask the frustration, and then the alcohol brought new frustrations. He wanted to become a minister again, but on the way to visit my father in the summer of 1974, a year before I was born, Frank showed up for an interview at a church in Rhode Island reeking of booze.

After that debacle, he and my father had their fiercest fight. "Why didn't we stop that terrible night?" my dad wrote in his diary on June 20. "One could make it the climax of a novel—the broken, dejected, and, alas, drunk father, reeling, screaming, moaning, asking for death, accusing his son of the grossest of perfidy." My father yelled that Frank needed to get ahold of himself and stop drinking. Frank yelled back that he was going to kill himself.

A few weeks later, my father wrote Frank a letter. It was kind and reasoned, but also pointed. "Remember, Dad, that whatever else can be said, I am one person, for whatever good or bad reasons, who shares your dreams, your dreams for you. I want so badly for you to have that 'other chance' that you dream of. And because I have those dreams for you, I can't control my subconscious rage when you sell yourself short, lose your self-confidence and control."

My grandfather responded a few days later, but in the meantime, something awful had happened. He had gotten so drunk that my grandmother had threatened to leave him. Now he was explaining to his son that he hadn't really been that intoxicated. He had just had a bit of champagne, a beer, and a scotch that someone else had brought to an event. My father had limited patience. He wrote in his diary: "My mind is filled with memories of his falling on the floor, cursing, fighting the winds, threatening, blackmailing—no less—suicide, and I should live my life for these memories? No, I have mine to lead."

He wrote back, countering his father's evasions and offering the way out: "There is an obvious solution. Stop Drinking." And then my father admonished his father for threatening to kill himself when visiting a month ago. "How a person who has used as his criterion of achievement service to others could even suggest such a termination of his own life boggles my mind."

For the next few years, my father's diary would go back to these events. He would grapple with them, wondering whether his own professional anxieties stemmed from his father's professional anxieties. Occasionally, he showed self-awareness that perhaps he should learn from his father and quit drinking himself. In July 1975, 20 days before I was born, he wrote about the fight from the year before. "Logically that should have done the trick and kept me off all booze for life. But the resentment was too much; I felt I needed—indeed I felt deserved—a 'boost' of some sort."

■

One day, after reading all these diary entries and documents again, I pulled out an old accordion-like bin where I had kept the letters I received as a young man. I wanted to see if there were any from my grandfather. But in the *T* section, one slid out that I thought I had long lost. It was from my father to me and dated the month I turned 21.

It started with something of an apology for him having turned his back on me when I was a baby struggling in the ICU. He had been making up for it, though, he said, ever since. He quoted Robert Nozick's *The Examined Life:* "There is no bond I know stronger than being a parent. Having children and raising them gives one's life substance. To have done so is at least to have done that." He then explained that talented young men often falter in life, but he didn't see that happening to me. My skills were dispersed in ways he envied. I was intrinsically happy. "Most important," he wrote, I had "beliefs and values." But, he added, "I do worry about your future." He knew that youthful promise is fraught. "Remember that as I look at your future I have all the tragedies around where promise turned sour." He worried that I would make reckless and impatient professional choices in my 20s. He worried that I would cast ambition aside and settle for a boring life out of "dislike for the Philistines of life, the compromises of it, the glitz of it."

He then added, "You still have a slight naivete about the harshness and pain of life, which might cause you to be blindsided at some point. Your older sister and I—it is no secret—have joked about your view that life just naturally arranges itself so conveniently for you. . . . People like to facilitate a handsome and charming young man, likewise a beautiful young lady. I recall the point Truman Capote made, when he said a good-looking man over six feet simply can't fathom the point of view of someone five foot two (like him)."

He continued. "Well, back to my starting point. That of the parent. We have to learn all over again to see the child as the adult as we begin our descent back into a form of childhood. . . . Obviously, when parents begin to use their children's successes as fungible substitutes for their own failures, the child first squirms and then rebels. No pain I ever felt in life—and there've been some big ones—equals that when I realized that my own father couldn't preserve a boundary between his own declining fortune and my rising ones."

He ended by returning to the desire he had had, so many years ago, to have a son. "I knew I wanted a son more than anything, and to the extent that I had intimations of a contrary sexuality, I was willing to sublimate them for life if need be to fulfill that ambition." Then he ended kindly, with sweet words about my mother, which was not his normal mode. "I know that your mother is equally rightly proud of all you've done and meant to people, and she gets tons of credit for softening the edges, inter alia, of some of those genes you may have got from me. And I don't mean that in any small sense."

My friends often ask me how I forgave my father. He caused

immense pain to my mother. He was an absent father for my younger sister. He put the three of us kids at serious physical risk. He threatened to kill himself and said I was to blame. He mooched money off me and used it to pay for sex. He exploited young men. He lived on the other side of the world. I could have let the relationship go.

I didn't, though, and maybe the reason is simple. A parent has one obligation to their children: unending love. They don't have to agree with every choice the child makes. They don't have to go to every track meet. They can demand things and refuse things. They can build a dam in a cold stream with the kid, or they can sit by the side and read. They can send a vague, loving note when their child turns 21, or a deep, incisive one. There's no blueprint and there's only one rule: the kids get to decide if the parent meets the standard. I was blessed by fate to have two parents who weren't meant to be with each other but who were each entirely devoted to me. That is worth forgiving a lot in exchange.

■

My life as a runner really dates back to one day: October 24, 1982, when at age seven I stood just past the Queensboro Bridge and handed my father a bottle of orange juice and a new pair of shoes. I remember standing there for a long while, which meant I would have seen Dick Beardsley and Alberto Salazar in the lead pack. I probably saw Bobbi Gibb gliding along, about 10 minutes behind my dad, en route to her fastest marathon. About 45 minutes after Gibb ran through, Sri Chinmoy would have passed by. It was the fourth and last time he ran the New York City Marathon, and he finished in four and a half hours. Up in Harlem, Tony Ruiz was watching the race with a hangover and cheering the runners on at Marcus Garvey Park.

I often wonder how my kids will look at my strange obsession. Ellis has never been drawn to running. Starting at age 12, though, he started going on arduous multi-day hikes with me in the White Mountains. And he inherited the gene for academic intensity. Most nights, I work until about 11 and then get up around 6 to start again. Ellis is always hard at work at his desk when I turn out my lights, and he's sometimes downstairs making coffee when I turn them back on.

In February 2024, I decided to enter a 10-mile race in Prospect Park. Zachary, now 13, had a rare weekend with almost no soccer scheduled, so, the day before the race, I asked whether he might want to come and join in the first 3.33-mile loop. We had gone on a few two-mile runs the previous weeks. He was playing a video game and said, offhandedly, "Sure." Later that day, he revised his goal: "Maybe, Dad, I'll try to run the whole thing," he said. I told him that this sounded a touch crazy, but that I'm not the kind of parent who'll say no to a crazy goal. I told him to be careful. I noted where on the course he could drop out and have the shortest walk home.

On race morning, we traveled together to the start. I began near the front, and he began near the middle of the pack. As I finished my last loop, I saw his familiar gray sweatshirt. I was sprinting to the line, and he yelled, "Go, Dad!" He was still in the race and had done almost seven miles. I crossed the line, and then we switched roles. "Go, Zachary," I yelled. He pushed onward and ended up running the last lap faster than the first two. He did the whole 10 miles and got a medal, which read "Cherry Tree 10-Miler," that he hung up in his room. The next year, he ran the race again, in a storm of freezing rain. I finished 30 minutes ahead of him the first year and 18 minutes ahead the second. That spring, he decided to join his school track team, at least on days he didn't have soccer practice in Queens. He ran a 4:58 mile, which is faster than I've run one in years.

James, meanwhile, has always loved to sprint, and he even trained a few times with Ruiz. In the spring of 2025, I started working as an informal running coach for James's elite age-10-and-11 soccer team. Each Monday, I would lead a big group of them in a mile run after they'd finished training on the field. James's mile time got better and better and was approaching 6 minutes. One day in early May, he declared that he wanted to get under that barrier. It was a dreary, rainy day and the track in Juniper Valley Park in Queens was soggy. I told James it wasn't going to be easy. But he said he was going to try. He ran the first half in 3:02 and then slowed and struggled to finish with a 6:09. He came to the line with a dark scowl and behind one of his teammates. I told him not to worry and sprinted off to encourage the team's central midfielder, who was trying to run 7:45. When I got back, James declared that he was going to do it again. I told him not to, but off he went. He ran alone, as his confused teammates watched and his unflappable coach called out the splits. He finished in 6:21. I felt worried that he had pushed himself too hard. But I also saw a little acorn out there; I can't say I wasn't a little proud. A few weeks later, he ran a 5:50.

We give our children our genes and our love, and we don't have any idea of what, in the end, they'll do with them. My grandfather scarred my father by trying to push him into sports; my father inspired me by taking me running around the block.

Maybe one of my sons will write a tell-all one day about the pressure his father put on him to be something he didn't want to be. Maybe they'll write about these days on the track or running around the park, in anger.

Or maybe they'll find that they love the sport too. One day, off in the future, if I'm lucky, I'll be handing one of them a gel on Atlantic Avenue or offering a new pair of shoes on the downside of the Queensboro Bridge. Maybe the passion will skip a generation, but I'll still end up drinking beet juice with my grandkids. My father led a deeply complicated and broken life. But he gave me many things, including the gift of running—a gift that opens the world to anyone who accepts it.

■

There are a lot of reasons why I run. I like the mental space it gives me. I like setting goals and trying to meet them. I like the feeling of my feet hitting the ground and the wind in my hair. I like to remember that I'm still alive, and that I survived my cancer. I think it makes me better at my job. But I run because of my father. Running connects me to my father; it reminds me of my father; and it gives me a way to avoid becoming my father.

The morning after my sisters and I arrived for my father's funeral in the Philippines, I put on my running shoes and headed up the hill above the villa. Batangas is a tough place to run: the roads don't have shoulders, there are dogs everywhere, jitneys screech by. That day, it was 90 degrees and humid. But I take pride in being able to run anywhere, and I wanted to understand this place and what he saw. I moved slowly up and past Banga Elementary School. Then I stopped. I wondered how far I was from the antipodal point of the planet from where my father grew up. If he had started digging a hole as a child in Oklahoma and gone all the way to the other side of the Earth, how far away would he have ended up from here?

I jogged back down to the house. Some of his friends from around the world had flown in, and it was time for the ceremony. He had always loved music, so I brought my guitar and played a short song I had composed for him. We all toasted his life, and the theme was similar, whether expressed by the Filipinos, the Americans, or the Europeans. No one had ever known anyone quite like Scott Thompson.

Afterward, I went up to his bedroom, with the curtains open to the lake and its imposing volcano. He had spent his days here, feeling the breeze, reading, typing out frantic emails. It was beautiful, and it comforted me to imagine him at peace here. I looked at his books, wondering which was the last one he read. I saw the painting of the Native American drummer that my father had taken from my childhood bedroom and then carried with him all over the world. And then I saw, on a shelf a few feet from the painting, a frame holding the story that I had written about my father many decades before.

A SPECIAL ACHIEVEMENT BY MY DAD

> I waited calmly at the sidelines of the New York City marathon in 1982 as I watched the front runners speed along at a terrific pace. I watched, and watched, and watched. Finally I saw my father. I called for him. He was among a mass of runners running at a steady pace. He ran over and I handed him his second pair of New Balance jogging shoes. He rapidly flipped off his sweaty, smelly sneakers and laced up the second pair. Then I handed him his bottle of orange juice that he had requested earlier. He

gulped it down while beginning to jog again and then tossed me the empty bottle. Only 6 miles left, he said between huffs and puffs.

We (a babysitter and I) drove to the finish line. It seemed like hours in the car because the traffic was so bad. Finally, we got there. After a little bit of time we located my father who had just run the best marathon of his life—3:00:17, just 18 seconds away from an under 3 hour marathon. He had a medal around his neck, for placing high in the 40 and older category. He said he never could have done [it] without my help, giving him a much needed pair of shoes and a reviving drink. He then handed me the medal and gave it to me.

The next day I went and got the paper, picked out the sports page about the marathon, located his name and circled it. Then I showed him the paper and ran and put it up in my room where it still is.

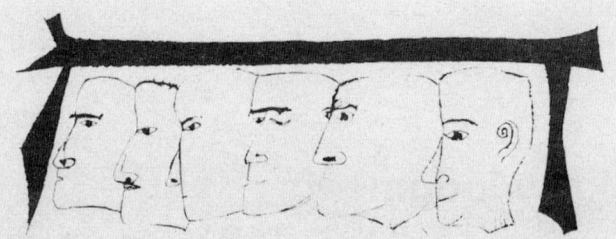

GOD HIMSELF, THE FATHER AND FASHIONER OF ALL THAT IS, OLDER THAN THE SUN OR THE SKY, GREATER THAN TIME AND ETERNITY AND ALL THE FLOW OF BEING, IS UNNAMEABLE BY ANY LAWGIVER, UNUTTERABLE BY ANY VOICE, NOT TO BE SEEN BY ANY EYE. BUT WE, BEING UNABLE TO APPREHEND HIS ESSENCE, USE THE HELP OF SOUNDS AND NAMES AND PICTURES, OF BEATEN GOLD AND IVORY AND SILVER, OF PLANTS AND RIVERS MOUNTAIN PEAKS AND TORRENTS, YEARNING FOR THE KNOWLEDGE OF HIM, AND IN OUR WEAKNESS NAMING ALL THAT IS BEAUTIFUL IN THIS WORLD AFTER HIS NATURE – JUST AS HAPPENS TO EARTHLY LOVERS TO THEM THE MOST BEAUTIFUL SIGHT WILL BE THE ACTUAL LINEAMENTS OF THE BELOVED. BUT FOR REMEMBRANCE' SAKE THEY WILL BE HAPPY IN THE SIGHT OF A LYRE, A LITTLE SPEAR, A CHAIR, PERHAPS, OR A RUNNING GROUND, OR ANYTHING IN THE WORLD THAT WAKENS THE MEMORY OF THE BELOVED. WHY SHOULD I FURTHER EXAMINE AND PASS JUDGEMENT ABOUT IMAGES? LET MEN KNOW WHAT IS DIVINE, LET THEM KNOW: THAT IS ALL. IF A GREEK IS STIRRED TO THE REMEMBRANCE OF GOD BY THE ART OF PHEIDIAS, AN EGYPTIAN BY PAYING WORSHIP TO ANIMALS, ANOTHER MAN BY A RIVER, ANOTHER BY FIRE – I HAVE NO ANGER FOR THEIR DIVERGENCES; ONLY LET THEM KNOW, LET THEM LOVE, LET THEM REMEMBER.

Closing Paragraph of Dissertatio VIII of Maximus of Tyre (1st Cent. A.D.)

Ben Shahn

Acknowledgments

I WANT TO START BY THANKING MY WIFE, DANIELLE, THE LOVE OF MY life. She was the first reader on the manuscript and the person who, for thirty years, has coped with this rather intense hobby of mine. Just thanks. I also want to thank my mother, for whom this manuscript was far from a simple read. This is a book about what I learned from him, but there's so much more that I learned from her. My two wonderful sisters, Phyllis and Heidi, both read an early version and offered corrections, details, adjustments, photographs, and deep insight. We each had our own relationship with our father, but we share deep love for each other. My eldest son, Ellis, was the second person to read the draft. As he said to me, "I learned a lot of interesting and new things about our family." In many ways, the project began on the flight back from the Philippines after my father's funeral when I started writing a letter to him, Zachary, and James about what Dad had meant to me. By the time I landed back at JFK, it was 5,000 words long. One of my central goals in life is to break the long string of Thompson fathers who have caused deep psychic angst for their children. I also want to thank two beloved women who are no longer with us but who were long members of my family: Florrie O'Riordan, who helped raise me, and Seeta Ramsaroop, who helped raise my boys. And I want to thank my stepfather, Marshall Moriarty, and my parents-in-law, Margaret and Martin Goldman, who were all early readers of the book.

It was not easy to settle on a structure for the book. It's probably wise for me to keep some of those deliberations secret. But I want to thank four people in particular. The first is my agent, Rafe Sagalyn, who came up with the initial theory of the book and who has encouraged and helped every step of the way. Then I was blessed to work closely with three extraordinary editors at Random House: Mark Warren, who eventually moved on to go and win a Pulitzer Prize for his own writing; Hilary Redmon, who eventually moved on to become the editorial director of Knopf, and Ben Greenberg, the editor in chief. I felt like a player on the peak Celtics coached by three hall-of-famers in succession. Each guided and improved the book in remarkable ways. And thank you to the rest of the wonderful team there: Milena Brown, Michael Hoak, Greg Kubie, Alison Rich, and Leila Tejani. An extra special thanks to Andy Ward, who has supported this project immensely from the very first day.

One of the virtues of spending my life in journalism is that I have a number of friends who offered incisive and constructive comments. I want to start with Corby Kummer, who went above and beyond the call of duty. He read five full different versions of the manuscript and offered terrific notes on each. (And, yes, Corby, you win: the sentence you kept putting back has survived to the final version.) Mark Boutros read an extremely early version and gave me confidence that I had something to work with. Vera Titunik edited the essay at *Wired* that helped inspire this book and offered her always astute comments on this manuscript. I was blessed to work with Vera at *The New Yorker* and at *Wired*. The only thing that would make me go back to the editing side of journalism would be if I knew I could work with her a third time. Larissa MacFarquhar—the Eliud Kipchoge of magazine writing—gave me the idea to begin the book with the recounting of the 2007 New York City Marathon. Pam McCarthy saved my journalism career by responding to that 3 A.M. email and offered wonderful insights on the manuscript. Her comments were given before I found the letter my father wrote me at age 21, but they had something rather in common with what he said too. Taylor Ho Bynum has been my closest friend since roughly the age of three, and he offered wisdom both on a written draft and on long hikes in the White Mountains. Roger Pasquier gave me a superb, detailed, and careful read. Josh Davis helped me think through the motivations of the characters I wrote about. Michael Joyner helped me make sure the science was accurate, and my training partner Carlos Garcia gave a detailed read as well. David Lavin at the Lavin Agency has been a terrific friend and partner for years and a great champion of this project. I also want to thank my other colleagues there who have supported this project: Ken Calway, Tom Gagnon, Cathy Hirst, Eliot Lavin, and Charles Yao. For the *Wired* essays that led to much of the early thinking for the book, I want to thank my editors John Gravois, Mark

Robinson, and Maria Streshinsky. ("Go deeper" was Maria's note on almost every draft.) And I want to thank the remarkable bosses I have had in my journalism career: Charlie Peters, Paul Glastris, Lincoln Caplan, Bob Cohn, Chris Anderson, Henry Finder, David Remnick, Roger Lynch, Anna Wintour, David Bradley, and Laurene Powell Jobs. And I'd like to give a special thank-you to Emily Locher, the very last friend to do a copy read of the book. She found errors that almost certainly would have made their way into print.

I want to thank the team at *The Atlantic* as well. Jeffrey Goldberg found time to offer brilliant insights and wisdom, even while dealing with the complexities of being included in the White House's Signal group chat. Scott Rosenfield and Ricki Harris helped me set up and manage the work schedule that made completing the manuscript possible, and Ricki was the first person at *The Atlantic* to read it through. I'm blessed too to work with them as well as with my indomitable Francesca Billington, who juggled one hundred projects with joy and alacrity. Megan Donohue read an early version and asked a hard but simple question: "Why is it better to be better at this?" Peter Mendelsund, Drew Campbell, and Laura Scofield gave me smart feedback on different cover designs. I also want to thank Peter Lattman and Steve McDermid for helping and encouraging me along. Anna Bross is our exceptional communications lead who will, no doubt, be expertly navigating its promotion by the time you read this. If it does have any readers, much of that will be due to the advice of Charles Duhigg, who has been as supportive a friend as one could ask for the past two decades. And thank you too to Mark Fortier, Ian Antonoff, Adam Benavides, and Marcus Plummer at Fortier Public Relations.

I called into service two remarkable former colleagues. Anna Goldwater Alexander selected and laid out all the photographs, and Sameen Gauhar checked all the facts. If there are errors, they are mine. If there are things that are accurate, it's because of Sameen. (She noticed, among other lovely errors, that I had gotten my own age wrong at one point in the manuscript and described an injury to my wrong Achilles.) And thank you to the astonishing Stuart Calderwood. He was my teammate on the Central Park Track Club and someone I always looked up to: the man has not missed a day of running for 38 years. Through good fortune and happenstance, he became Random House's copy editor for the book. Among other things, he gave me the information that allowed me to turn a hypothetical joke about white-collar crime into a definitive fact.

I want to thank the people who agreed to be interviewed by me during this process or who responded to my fact-checking queries: Gary Allen, Margaret Angell, Neftalem Araia, Lisa Barrett, Trevor Bayliss, Zack Beavin, Tracy Bennett, Chrissy Bergren, Michael Blanton, Arthur Brooks, Leila Burr, Monal Choksi, Jesse Cody, Yung Cohen, Andy Cowgill, Josh Cox, Harita Davies, David Epstein, Jason German, Ryan Hall, Joe Holder, Michael Holder, Rachel Hyland, Kilian Jornet, Michael Joyner, Alan Katz, Meb Keflezighi, Bob Kempainen, Brett Kirby, Matt Kneller, Vin Lananna, Charlie Lawrence, Desiree Linden, Emily Locher, John Luce, Chris Lundstrom, Steve Magness, Dave McGillivray, Brian Mendonca, Maryam Naghavi, Aaron Padilla, Daniel Pink, Sanjay Rawal, David Remnick, Knox Robinson, Lisa Rosenbaum, Alan Rouvez, Peter Sagal, Dov Seidman, Jon Stableford, John Strudwick, Ken Weisbrode, Rick West, and Greg Whitmore.

I want to thank friends in the industry who have supported

me along the way, including Sean Hyland at New Balance, Matthew Kneller at Nike, Lucas Maher at Puma, Nnenna Lynch at New York Road Runners, Ben Morrow at Miler Running, and Matt Taylor at Tracksmith. And I want to thank the friends who pulled me along or otherwise supported me in the races described in the book, including David Alm, Shawn Bubany, Ali Burnes, Judson Cake, Corey Henry, Ford McElroy, Jack Mulvaney, Alan Ruben, Leigh Anne Sharek, and Harsha Thirumurthy.

I also want to of course thank Suprabha Beckjord, Bobbi Gibb, Julia Lucas, Tony Ruiz, and Michael Westphal. And a special thanks to Steve Finley. When Danielle read the final version she said, "He's kind of the hero of this, isn't he?"

The person I wish I could have sent the book to is of course my father. The last email I ever received from him encouraged me to, one day, "write great memoirs." He added, "I'd love to stick around to read it, and won't discourage total if sometimes painful candor."

Dad, you weren't easy. But I love you.

Photograph Credits

All photographs are courtesy of the author except as noted below.

    PAGE 242: © 2025 Estate of Ben Shahn/Licensed by VAGA at Artists Rights Society (ARS), NY.

INSERT

    PAGE 1: David Paz

    PAGE 3, bottom: Courtesy of Phillips Academy, Andover

    PAGE 4: David Hashim

    PAGE 6: Fred Kaplan/Sports Illustrated via Getty Images

    PAGE 7: AP Photo/Charlie Riedel

    PAGE 8, top: srichinmoyultraphoto.com

    PAGE 9: Peter Frank Edwards/Redux

    PAGE 10: © Stephen Russell Shilling, used with permission

    PAGE 11: Sarah Stafford

    PAGE 12, top: Image courtesy of NIKE, Inc.

    PAGE 14, top: Courtesy of Christina Odendahl

    PAGE 14, bottom: David Hashim

    PAGE 15: David Hashim

    PAGE 16: Image courtesy of NIKE, Inc.

    PHOTO EDITOR: Anna Goldwater Alexander

ABOUT THE AUTHOR

NICHOLAS THOMPSON is the CEO of *The Atlantic,* an American magazine founded in 1857, which earned the top honor for magazines, General Excellence, at the National Magazine Awards in 2022, 2023, and 2024. Before joining *The Atlantic,* he was the editor in chief of *Wired* and an editor at *The New Yorker.* He has long been a competitive runner; in 2021, he set the American record for men 45+ in the 50K race. In 2025, he became the top-ranked runner in the world in his age group for the 50-mile run. He lives in Brooklyn, New York, with his wife and three sons.

nickthompson.com
Instagram: @nxthompson
X: @nxthompson
Facebook.com/nxthompson
Linkedin.com/in/nicholasxthompson

ABOUT THE TYPE

This book was set in Scala, a typeface designed by Martin Majoor in 1991. It was originally designed for a music company in the Netherlands and then was published by the international type house FSI FontShop. Its distinctive extended serifs add to the articulation of the letterforms to make it a very readable typeface.